YOGA

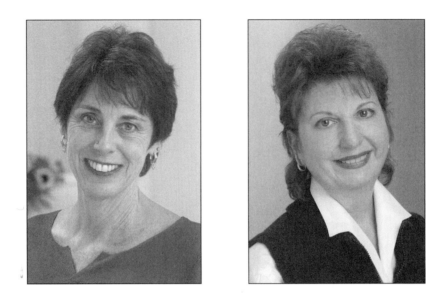

About the Authors

Elise Browning Miller, M.A. is a Senior Certified Iyengar Yoga teacher from Palo Alto who has been teaching yoga since 1976. She has studied numerous times with B.K.S. Iyengar and Geeta Iyengar in India. As a founding director of the California Yoga Center in Mountain View, CA, Elise teaches classes, has a private practice specializing in back and sports-related injuries, and teaches workshops and retreats around the world. Elise has successfully used yoga to minimize the effects of her own scoliosis and sees clients privately with scoliosis and other back related problems. She has published numerous articles on scoliosis and other yoga related subjects in *Yoga Journal* and other national magazines and has recently released the new video and booklet, *Yoga for Scoliosis*. Elise is a board member and treasurer of the California Yoga Teachers Association and also a faculty member at the Iyengar Yoga Institute of San Francisco.

Carol Blackman, M.A., is a journalist who writes about health and fitness, business on the Internet, and travel destinations. She is a co-author of *Yoga: Anytime, Anywhere* and two travel guide books: *Way To Go! Shopping in San Francisco* and *Best Bay Area Bargains*. Carol spent fourteen years as a reporter, columnist, editor and manager with two daily newspapers in the San Francisco Bay area and has written feature stories for a variety of specialty magazines.

YOGA

ANYTIME, ANYWHERE

Elise Browning Miller
and
Carol Blackman

Llewellyn Publications
St. Paul, Minnesota

SECOND EDITION
First printing, 2004

Cover design: Ellen Dahl
Cover photograph © 2004: Geoff Nilsen
Cover model: Elise Browning Miller
Editing and project management for second edition: Sandy Leuthner
Editing and book design: Christine Snow
Additional editing: Amy Rost
Additional book design: Donna Burch
Interior photos © 1998: Sam Forencich
Author photographs © 2004: Geoff Nilsen
Photos for second edition in Chapter 9 and Chapter 14 © 2004: Geoff Nilsen
Photos in Chapter 3 and on pages 176–180 © 1998: Elise Browning Miller
Line art illustrations © 1998: Kerigwen

Library of Congress Cataloging-in-Publication Data

Miller, Elise Browning, 1948-
  [Life is a Stretch]
  Yoga: anytime, anywhere / Elise Browning Miller ; Carol Blackman.—2nd ed.
    p. cm.
  Rev. ed. of: Life is a stretch.
  Includes bibliographical references and index.
  ISBN 0-7387-0635-3
  1. Hatha yoga. 2. Stretching exercises. I. Blackman, Carol, 1948- II. Title

RA781.7M53 2004
613.7'046—dc22

2004048600

Llewellyn Worldwide does not participate in, endorse, or have any authority or responsibility concerning private business transactions between our authors and the public. All mail addressed to the author is forwarded but the publisher cannot, unless specifically instructed by the author, give out an address or phone number.

Any Internet references contained in this work are current at publication time, but the Publisher cannot guarantee that a specific location will continue to be maintained. Please refer to the Publisher's website for links to authors' websites and other sources.

The practices, techniques, and stretches described in this book should not be used as an alternative to professional medical treatment. This book does not attempt to give any medical diagnosis, treatment, prescription, or suggestion for medication in relation to any human disease, pain, injury, deformity, or physical condition.

The authors and publisher of this book are not responsible in any manner whatsoever for any injury which may occur through following the instructions contained herein. It is recommended that before beginning the stretches and techniques, you consult with your physician to determine whether you are medically, physically, and mentally fit to undertake this course of practice.

Llewellyn Publications
A Division of Llewellyn Worldwide, Ltd.
P.O. Box 64383, Dept. 0-7387-0635-3
St. Paul, MN 55164-0383

 Printed in the United States of America on recycled paper

Acknowledgments

Elise Browning Miller

To my father, G. Tyler, who always gave me the encouragement to follow my dream and taught me to live life with an open heart.

To my mother, Elise, for always being there.

To my yoga teacher, the Honorable B. K. S. Iyengar, for his inspiration and guidance as a teacher and artist for whom I have unlimited respect and gratitude for his willingness to share it with us all.

Carol Blackman

To Sandy Leuthner, our editor/mentor at Llewellyn, and to our readers who are helping themselves to healthier and happier lives.

CONTENTS

Dear Reader

Yoga may not be on your daily list of things to do. Yet.

Five years ago, when my friend Elise and I wrote *Life Is a Stretch: Easy Yoga, Anytime, Anywhere*, folks were just beginning to use yoga (we called it yoga-style "stretching") as a part of their regular fitness routines. Instead of needing to study traditional yoga by taking a class, we gave readers an easy way to fit "yoga stretching" into everyday life—yoga stretching at your computer, yoga stretching when you are on a plane trip, and yoga stretching before taking a run or long walk. I promised readers then that they would not have to learn to put their legs behind their heads or get

Ph.D.'s in Eastern philosophy. And I am keeping those promises.

However, since writing *Life Is a Stretch*, interest in traditional styles of yoga practice has increased tremendously. Many people do take classes. But even the reader who practices yoga in regular classes can benefit from fitting yoga stretching into everyday life.

To include more traditional yoga instruction, we have revised *Life Is a Stretch* by adding two new chapters: Chapter 9, "Strengthen and Stretch with Classic Yoga Poses;" and Chapter 14, "Create Your Own Yoga Practice." The result is this new edition, *Yoga: Anytime, Anywhere*.

For readers who are new to yoga, we start with explaining what yoga means and we list the many benefits. We talk about beginning a "Yoga Stretching Program" and tell you how the book is organized and what equipment you will need.

For readers who have some experience with yoga, the step-by-step instructions on how to correctly do the poses are a good reminder of how to practice yoga outside of class, and can help you to maintain a solid home practice. For the more traditional poses in Chapter 9, we lead you through the process of starting with a prop (a chair, a block) and working up to practicing these poses in the traditional way. In Chapter 14, we give you suggested routines to improve your health and vitality every day. And we have updated our resources section with current books, experts, and yoga connections to help you enjoy your commitment to your personal yoga plan.

It is easy to learn how to breathe, stretch and relax throughout your day. We wrote *Yoga: Anytime, Anywhere* to give you even more benefits from your yoga practice. Let's get started.

Cheers,
Carol Blackman

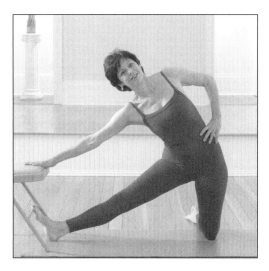

c h a p t e r   1

Learn About Yoga Stretching

The desire to stretch is a natural impulse. Cats and dogs stretch repeatedly during the day whenever they feel stiff. Humans too can get great benefits from knowing how to stretch and breathe for stress reduction and a sense of feeling youthful, alive and more vital.

Yoga stretching can be very a practical and useful tool in your life. You don't have to go off to India for months and meditate. You don't have to stand on your head, although that can be beneficial. As a matter of fact, the stretching practiced as yoga poses is a basic physical need for people of all ages and all levels of fitness.

What Is Yoga?

Let us start with a simple definition. Yoga is a 3,000-year-old Eastern discipline from India that incorporates the physical, mental, and spiritual parts of one's being. Yoga means union, so you are uniting the body, mind, and spirit. For this book, we are focusing on the use of Hatha yoga, which concentrates on the physical. This is one of the many branches of yoga practice. We will use breathing, yoga postures, and relaxation techniques to improve your flexibility, balance, strength, and endurance.

Even though we are focusing on the physical postures and breathing in this book, we know that traditional yoga includes mental concentration that ultimately leads to the practice of meditation. Yoga philosophy was systematized and first recorded some 2,000 years ago by the Sage Patanjali in the *Yoga Sutras*, a work acknowledged as the authoritative text of yoga. Patanjali describes yoga as the method by which the restless mind is calmed and the energy is directed into constructive channels. He felt that the right means are just as important as the end view. The methods to still the mind are organized into eight stages of yoga. This is known as the eight-fold path or *asatanga*. The eight-fold path includes:

- *Yama*: moral restraint
- *Niyama*: personal discipline
- *Asana*: posture
- *Pranayama*: rhythmic breath control
- *Pratyahara*: control of the senses
- *Dharana*: concentration
- *Dyhana*: meditation
- *Samadhi*: enlightenment

There are many styles of yoga that have come to the United States. The type of yoga we are using for this book is the Iyengar style. The Iyengar (I´yen´gär) style of yoga is named after Mr. B. K. S. Iyengar of India, who authored many books including *Light On Yoga* (George Allen & Unwin, 1966) and *Light On Pranayama* (Crossroad Publishing, 1981). This system of stretching emphasizes the details of how to do the poses correctly, with proper alignment, and how to prevent injury. He adapted the traditional yoga poses by using props, such as a wall or a chair, to make it possible for novices to get benefits from these poses. Also, he created his style to help people with specific physical problems. This makes it a very practical system. Because the instructions for our poses include awareness of detail and mental concentration, the practice of the Iyengar style will, in fact, involve all of the stages of the eight-fold path of yoga.

Simple Stretching vs. Yoga

When you are doing yoga postures, there is an awareness of the breath and a focusing of the mind. This process becomes as important as the end result. For example, in stretching, the goal may be to touch your toes. When you do a yoga pose, you may touch your toes, but you are focusing your attention on body alignment, muscle tension, and breath awareness. It becomes much more than just a physical exercise. This is how you start to learn how to reduce stress.

Yoga Stretching Benefits

Yoga stretching is definitely in the mainstream of exercise these days. Since the 1970s, many celebrities have been practicing yoga. The list includes entertainers such as the Beatles and actress Jane Fonda and sports stars such as Kareem Abdul Jabar. Physical therapists, sports physiologists, and medical doctors are now recommending it for health benefits. For example, Dr. Dean Ornish, a world-renowned cardiologist, uses yoga as part of his popular program to reverse heart disease. Here is a list of the benefits of making yoga stretching a part of your regular routine:

- Feel more youthful and look it
- Increase vitality and energy
- Cope more effectively with stress
- Release muscle tightness
- Improve posture
- Increase flexibility
- Develop strength and stamina
- Help with back problems
- Improve suppleness of the spine
- Keep organs, glands, and nerves in working order
- Improve digestion and elimination
- Enhance the body's immune response
- Therapeutically work to improve a variety of medical problems
- Improve circulation
- Decrease cholesterol and blood sugar levels
- Encourage weight loss
- Think more clearly
- Help with concentration
- Calm the mind

- Learn to relax
- Bring more balance, awareness, and joy into your life

Yoga is the perfect exercise for anyone who feels stiff. The only goal is to feel more flexible than when you started. And it is never too late to start. Some people have started yoga in their sixties or older and have found many benefits.

Posture and Back Care

Not only does your mood dramatically affect your posture, but conversely, your posture affects your mood. Remember a moment when you were depressed and look at your posture in your mind's eye. Now remember a time when you were totally joyful and excited. Your posture was probably a lot more open and energetic. Aligning your posture has a positive effect on your mental as well as your physical state.

Posture can be affected by muscular imbalances that have developed over time. Chronically poor posture can lead to significant back problems. Many people come to yoga because the yoga poses help to strengthen and stretch the muscles that affect posture.

When your posture is poor, your bone structure is not aligned and centered. As a result, your muscles do all the work to hold you up rather than sharing the job with the alignment of your bones. One example is when your head gets in front of the rest of your body. As a result of your head being in front, your shoulders round and move forward while your chest sinks. Your shoulder muscles (particularly the trapezius muscles) are overworking constantly, tensing to try to keep your head up. This also tenses your neck.

A tight muscle is not a strong muscle. Usually, it is a weak muscle. Each of your joints is controlled by at least two sets of muscles: the flexors, which bend the joint; and the extensors, which straighten it. Also, a number of joints have rotator muscles that twist and rotate the bones. These flexors, extensors, and rotators need to be in balance, but often the muscles are out of balance. For example, your flexors might be tighter and shorter than your extensors, causing unequal forces that make the joint weaker and more unstable. This will affect the bones, which will then be out of alignment. Through yoga, we begin to balance our muscle groups, and through awareness and effort, align our bones. Then muscles will not have to work overtime.

Yoga postures create movement and more flexibility of the spine, which help alleviate back pain. The discs, or thick pads of cartilage that separate adjacent vertebrae, do not get direct blood supply. Discs are dependent on a sponge-like action for attracting and absorbing nutrients from adjacent tissues. Flexing and extending the spine helps to bring this blood supply into your discs, thereby preventing degenerative disc disease, such as bulging and ruptured discs. The movement principle of yoga is "spreading" or creating space, "squeezing" or compressing liquids, muscles, and/or organs in that area and "soaking" or allowing blood and fluids to flow back in and cleanse that area.

Yoga also helps you to maintain the four natural curves of your body. The curve in your neck (cervical spine) and lower back (lumbar spine) are concave (curve in). The curve in your midback (thoracic) and sacrum (five fused vertebrae in the pelvis) are convex (round out). These natural curves are shock absorbers for the impact of gravity and normal movement in your everyday life. Curves that are too extreme, such as a rounded thoracic spine (kyphosis) or an extreme lumbar curve (lordosis), will often cause back pain. Yoga can help return these curves to a normal state. Consult your physician if you suffer from long-term back pain.

Beginning a Yoga Stretching Program

Tightness is not something that happens to us; we do it to ourselves. Once you start to stretch, your body is eager to let go of the tension it has been holding for years. You can break your old habit of simply running from one task to the next. Choosing to do these stretches during your regular routines can help you to slow down. The more often you do these poses, the more benefits you will receive.

Yoga is a gentle approach to exercise. **However, before starting any new exercise program, and especially if you have any special health concerns, you should consult your doctor first.**

We have designed the routines in this book to help most people, even if you have not maintained another regular exercise program.

Here are some general guidelines before starting your program:

- "No pain, no gain" does not apply to yoga; performing the stretches in these routines should not hurt

- Do not push yourself; find your own "edge" and stay there until your skill increases

- Try to practice on an empty stomach; at least do not start immediately after a meal

- Wear comfortable clothing that allows freedom of movement

- Do not do inversion postures during menses

- Choose a special place to do your yoga that is a clean, quiet location free from distractions and interruptions; let the answering machine take over

- Try to be consistent—the more you practice, the better you will feel

- Allow yourself to return to yoga if you lapse in your practice; no guilt trips
- Even though a new pose may be challenging, remind yourself to stay relaxed
- You may want to use a mirror in the beginning to gain more awareness of alignment; then see if you can become more aware from the inside without it
- Be persistent and energetic, but at the same time be gentle and non-violent
- Don't compare yourself with anyone else—yoga is non-competitive
- Move at your own pace and remember we all learn at different rates
- Forget the "shoulds"; listen to your body and your own inner voice
- The breath is the key; it helps you to feel and listen rather than to have expectations; it's the link between the body and the mind

As with any exercise program, never push your body beyond your capability and never stretch beyond your comfort level. We will teach you how to use your breath to expand your stretch for each pose.

How This Book Is Organized

You can do yoga anytime and anywhere. The yoga poses in this book are planned for different locations and situations so that you can see how you can put these stretches into your daily routine. Beyond what we are showing, you can be creative with where you practice your routines. Also, anyone can benefit from the breathing exercises in all of the chapters right away.

Here is how the book is organized:

Each chapter starts with breathing exercises, then gives instructions for appropriate stretching exercises, and ends with a relaxation process. Recording the relaxation sessions on an audio tape and listening to them on a small recorder with earphones may help you to enjoy the relaxation process more.

To follow the breathing, stretching, and relaxation for any chapter, it should take approximately twenty to thirty minutes once you learn the routine. If you are short on time, you can do just a few of the stretches and the relaxation.

The stretches become a little more challenging as you progress through the book.

Chapter 2 teaches you how to breathe and practice correct posture.

Chapters 3 through 13 focus on particular problems or body conditions.

Chapter 9 shows you how to progress from using a prop (a chair or a block) to practicing classic poses in the traditional way.

Chapter 14 lists poses to create routines to help stretch and strengthen a particular body area.

The Sanskrit names (in parenthesis) are given for some of the more traditional yoga poses.

In each chapter, we tell you if you might need to find a pillow or blanket or belt to use as simple equipment. This information will be marked "Equipment Note."

We have also added our own personal notes to tell you a little more about the benefits or give you extra advice.

More importantly, watch for our notes of caution when a particular stretch or routine is not recommended for individuals with certain conditions. They will be marked "Caution."

When you get familiar with all of the stretches, you may design your own program for your needs. If you were to use all of the stretches, you would have a total program.

We often separate our exercise program from the rest of our lives or set our goals so high that we can never reach them. We know that taking a class on yoga, in addition to your daily stretching, can enhance your health even more. However, if you don't have time to go to class, you can still fit yoga into your life. It is just as beneficial to do ten to twenty minutes of stretching per day as to cram it into a ninety-minute class once a week.

Equipment Needed

We suggest that you use some simple yoga equipment. Suggested resources are given in the back of the book for help in finding them. However, it is not necessary to buy anything special at first. Use things in your home, such as books, firm blankets, chairs, sofas, beds, counters, and stairways. You can also apply your poses in other places, such as while running errands or enjoying recreational activities.

If you want to use traditional yoga equipment, we suggest the following:

- Yoga sticky mat
- Yoga belt
- Three yoga blankets (firm)
- Yoga bolster
- Two yoga blocks

The most important of these is a sticky mat to help with slippery floors. If you do not use official yoga blankets, make sure the ones you do use are firm, preferably made of wool or cotton, to ensure you have enough support. If you don't have yoga blocks, use books with the approximate dimensions of 2"x5"x8". Watch for equipment notes at the beginning of each chapter to give you a list of equipment needed for those series of stretches.

Getting Started

We want you to use this practical guide to help put yoga into your day. The first step is learning how to use your breath and practice correct posture. So, let us begin with learning how to breathe in Chapter 2.

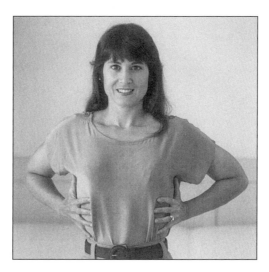

chapter 2

So You Think You Can Breathe

Do you ever feel . . .

. . . you are so stressed or anxious that you are about to burst? Do you hold your breath when a stressful situation comes up? Or even when you're exercising? Maybe you have felt your heart and breath racing during fearful or emotional situations.

When we become stressed, our attention is focused on external things. It may sound funny, but we often forget to breathe. Holding our breath creates more tension in our body and sends stress signals to the central nervous system. This can make your blood pressure rise and may cause you to feel out of breath.

Conscious breath control, or *pranayama*, is an important part of yoga. It helps to reduce stress and create more relaxation in your life. When we unconsciously breathe during a normal day, the volume and quality of breath depends on our physical and emotional state. It requires no thought or concentration.

On the other hand, with pranayama, we learn to control the breath through mental focus, therefore increasing the "prana," or life-force energy within us.

Also, by regulating the breath, we calm the entire nervous system. It has often been stated that the breath is the link between the body and the mind. By linking conscious breathing with the movements of stretching, we develop better concentration and stay in the present. Also, the movements become easier.

The diaphragm is a sheet of muscle at the base of the chest cavity that regulates the volume of the breath. Because the diaphragm is intimately linked to the spinal column, holding your breath and tightening the diaphragm will contract and strain the spine. Because the ribs are also attached to the spine, the upward and downward movements of respiration indirectly massage and lubricate the vertebral joints.

In this chapter, you will learn simple breathing exercises that you can do anytime you feel stressed or tired, whether sitting, standing, or lying on your back. You can use these techniques to prepare for any situation that makes you feel anxious or to calm you down after a stressful event. Take a few minutes to breathe and you will feel renewed and more relaxed. We promise that you will have more energy to continue whatever you are doing.

In yoga there is a saying: "The mouth is for eating, the nose is for breathing." Therefore, in yoga breathing, we normally breathe through the nose. By breathing through the nose, we can control and slow the breath down much more easily. In the beginning, it may feel unnatural, but as you practice, you will feel more calm and relaxed.

✔ **Equipment Note:** None required.

Breathing

Parts to the Complete Breath

When we are stressed, many of us become shallow chest breathers or belly breathers. We rarely use our full lung capacity, utilizing only a third of our lungs. This Complete Breath exercise will enhance your oxygen intake and teach you to breathe into three areas: the diaphragm, the chest, and the upper chest. In the upper chest, the lungs come to a point above the collarbone, and we rarely breathe into this area.

In order to get in touch with each of these three areas, we will go through each one in turn. We will breathe fully into each part. Then, we will combine the three parts into a Complete Breath. You can learn this breath standing up, sitting in a chair, or lying on your back.

> **Part one:** Place one hand at your belly where your diaphragm is located and the other at your lower back. (See Figure 2.1.) Begin to inhale, taking a long, deep breath through your nose, bringing the breath down to the belly and lower back, letting your hands expand in both directions. Now, imagine this is a balloon filling out in all directions. Now exhale and your diaphragm will relax, letting the belly soften, releasing the breath. Repeat this exercise three times or more.

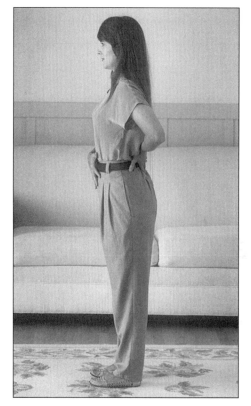

Figure 2.1
Part one of the Complete Breath

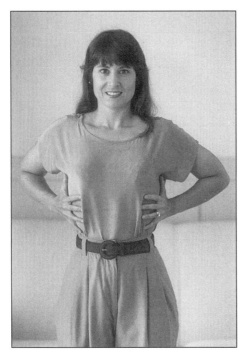

Figure 2.2
Part two of the Complete Breath

Part two: Bring the hands to the rib cage, below the breastbone, with the hands wrapping around the ribs, fingertips facing each other. Be sure that the heels of your hands are in line with the sides of your body. Your fingers should not touch in front. (See Figure 2.2.) Take a deep breath into this area, breathing into the ribs, feeling your hands expand from the sides to the front. It's important to feel the sides of the ribs expand first, letting the breath continue to expand to the front. Repeat three times or more.

Part three: Place your hands on your upper chest, with your fingers resting on your collarbone. (See Figure 2.3.) Take a deep breath and feel the upper chest expand, imagining the air filling the lungs all the way up to the collarbone. Exhale slowly and release the air, relaxing the upper chest. Repeat three times or more.

Three Parts of the Complete Breath with Arm Movements

Now you are ready to link these three parts together with arm movements. The arm movements help you breathe more fully into each area. You will now take one Complete Breath, inhaling in three parts: one third into the belly, one third into the rib cage, and one third into the upper chest. This helps to create equal ratio of breath into each area. You need to practice this standing with your feet parallel and hip-width apart, with your arms at your sides.

Remember: This is *one* breath being divided into three parts, pausing for a second between each part.

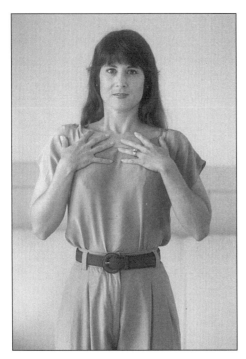

Figure 2.3
Part three of the Complete Breath

Part one: As you inhale one third of your breath into your belly, bring your arms straight out in front of you up to shoulder level. (See Figure 2.4.) Pause and feel the air in your belly.

Part two: As you inhale the second third of the breath into the rib cage, bring your arms out to your sides, keeping them at shoulder level. (See Figure 2.5.) As you pause to feel the air in your rib cage, stretch out through the arms and fingers, spreading the shoulder blades from the spine and feeling the ribs expanding out to the sides.

Part three: Inhale the last third of the breath into the upper chest and collarbone area, lifting the arms overhead, with the palms facing each other. (See Figure 2.6, page 16.) Pause and stretch up through the arms to coax the air into the upper chest.

Now slowly exhale all of the air, releasing the breath from top to bottom, and bringing the arms back down to the sides.

Repeat five times to practice equalizing the breath.

Some people find that they run out of breath when they get to the upper chest. If this happens to you, just practice taking less breath into the first two areas.

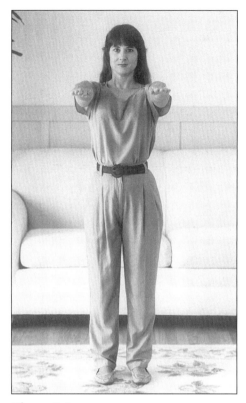

Figure 2.4
Part one: breathe into the belly with arms in front

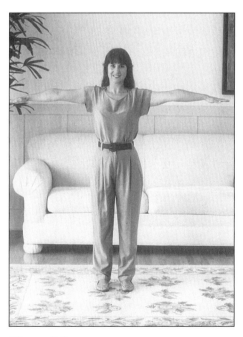

Figure 2.5
Part two: breathe into the ribs with arms out to your sides

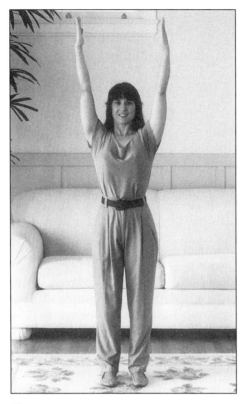

Figure 2.6
Part three: breathe into upper chest
while lifting arms overhead

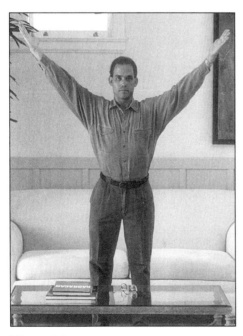

Figure 2.7
The Complete Breath in one
continuous movement

Complete Breath

Now that you have become familiar with breathing into the three distinct areas with arm movements, it is time to put it all together into one Complete Breath. With one continuous movement of the arms in the same pattern, you will practice taking one continuous, long deep breath.

Bring your arms down by your sides with your palms facing out. As you inhale, begin to bring your arms up from your sides to waist level, filling your belly with air. As you bring the arms up to chest level, continue to breathe, bringing the air into the rib cage. Now as you lift your arms overhead, palms facing together, allow the breath to flow into the upper chest, creating a flow of breath from bottom to top. (See Figure 2.7.) Slowly exhale, releasing the breath from top to bottom, bringing the arms down to the sides. Repeat three times.

As you become more comfortable with the Complete Breath, you can practice this with or without the arm movements, standing in line at the bank, sitting at your desk, or lying in bed.

Hissing Breath (Ujjayi)

Here is a breathing technique that will energize and calm you. This sounds like a contradiction but through years of practice, yoga experts discovered that this particular technique increases your oxygen intake, expands your mental capacity to focus, and calms the nervous system.

You will learn to create a slight hissing sound. The sound can serve as a reminder to breathe consciously in stressful situations. You can practice this standing, sitting, or lying down. Take a few normal breaths to become aware of your breathing.

> Close your mouth and drop the chin toward the chest to partially close the glottal region of the trachea. Allow the chin to create a slight pressure in the throat.

> As you inhale through your nose, begin to feel as if you are pulling the breath directly into the throat, creating the hissing sound called *Ujjayi* breath. Even though you are breathing in through the nose, the hissing will be made by a partial closure of your throat.

> On the exhalation, feel a sensation of pushing the breath out from that same area. You may want to make the sound as loud as you can to remind yourself to use this breath. In the beginning, it's easier to hear more sound on your exhalation. You may think you sound like Darth Vader and that's good. There is a feeling of filtering the breath in and out. As you practice this breath, you can make a quieter sound that only you hear. Now let that sensation spread throughout your body.

> Practice five to ten more conscious breaths in and out. Now bring the chin back up. Eventually, you will be able to create this hissing sound without dropping your chin.

✔ **Elise's Note:** I used this breath before the delivery of my son. It kept me calm and focused. After you learn the feeling of constricting your breath, see if you can bring the breath down to your collarbone area and breathe more softly so you won't constrict your throat so much. This will reduce the constriction in your face and brain.

✔ **Carol's Note:** Try this when you are caught in a traffic jam. You're not going anywhere and it will help to accept the obvious.

Now that you have learned to breathe, you are ready to add some yoga stretches into your life to help you cope with everyday stress. As we present a list of stretches for every situation, we will tell you to breathe along with the stretches. The Complete Breath as a whole or in parts can be used anytime, anywhere to reduce stress and remind you to relax. Since you can hear it, the hissing breath is a great way to remember to breathe during yoga stretches.

Now let's learn how to check your posture.

Posture

Palm Tree Pose (Tadasana)

Posture: Kick your shoes off. Stand up straight with your feet placed hip-width apart. Begin to notice your posture. Are you leaning on one foot more than another? Sway from side to side without falling over. See if you can bring the weight equally on both feet.

Balance: Is your weight on the balls of your feet, ready to spring into the next project? If so, see if you can bring the weight back into your heels, so you feel aligned from your head to your heels.

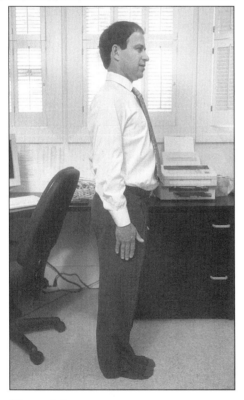

Figure 2.8
Palm Tree Pose

Feel your heels descend down into the floor as if they were roots stabilizing you. In yoga, this pose is called Palm Tree Pose. (See Figure 2.8, page 18.)

This position emphasizes grounding the feet into the floor, signifying roots of a tree spreading into the earth. Lift the toes for a moment, let them stretch and breathe and then bring them down to the floor without scrunching them up. Those toes have been captured by shoes for a lifetime so don't get discouraged if you can't bring them down without curling them. It is possible to have toes that function individually rather than as a unit. The legs, being the trunk of the tree, must be strong, with thigh muscles lifted, giving support to the rest of the body.

Shoulders: Are your shoulders lifted and your chest sunken? Inhale and lift and tense the shoulders, bringing them to the ears. Now exhale, letting your shoulders and shoulder blades drop down away from your ears. If your shoulders are particularly tense, you can practice this a few times. No longer do you have to carry the world on your shoulders.

Head: Is your head in front of your body, perhaps projecting into the future with your brain going full steam ahead? If so, see if you can align your head with the rest of the body, bringing the back of the head in line with your back. Is your jaw jutting forward, ready to put the next idea into action? If so, let go of your "To Do" list for now.

Breathe and feel an imaginary plum line from the crown of your head down through your ears, shoulders, and all the way down through your hips and ankles to your heels. (See Figure 2.9.)

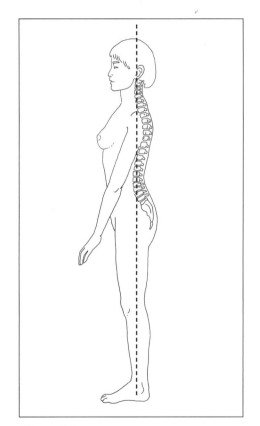

Figure 2.9
To help obtain proper posture shown here, feel an imaginary plumb line going down from the crown of your head all the way through your body

Once you have checked your posture alignment, you are ready to begin breathing, stretching, and relaxing. At first, you may want to look in a mirror from the side to check out your alignment since in the beginning it's hard to know where you are in space. After you've done this a few times, you can eliminate the mirror since you will start to see and feel it from the inside.

You are now ready to take a look at all of our specific stretches that apply to typical life situations. Find the first one that applies to you and get started.

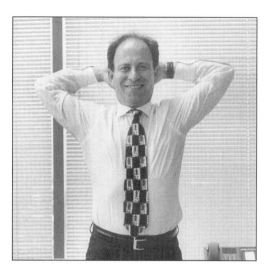

chapter 3

Stretch in the Office

Do you ever feel . . .

. . . you have so much work to do, you are about to scream? If you have been concentrating on any task for a period of time, you are probably holding tension in your neck, shoulders, and upper back. Your eyes resemble the street map of any large metropolitan area. Over time, the tension builds beyond what feels normal and your muscles are really screaming for relief.

Most of us are much more sedentary in our jobs than our ancestors were. A century ago, physical labor was far more prevalent.

Today, you can sit virtually motionless at the computer for eight hours or more. The only exercise is repetitive hand and wrist movements, which can cause wrist tendinitis and carpal tunnel syndrome. You feel you are too busy to do the very activities that would help you unwind and relax, and you can become emotionally drained.

This chapter will show you stretches you can do in twenty minutes to release the tension in your neck, shoulders, and upper back and also help to realign the body. When your head gets ahead of your shoulders, the muscles overwork and carry all of the weight. The alignment of the head and spine uses the bone structure to support the head on the neck and shoulders, which can also lead to lower back tension.

These stretches do not need to be done in a particular order or even all in one session. You may scatter them one or two at a time throughout the day. Notice where you are tense and do the stretches that address that particular area. Give yourself "an energy break." Some people use a timer to alert them when it is time to take a stretch break. These stretches can be done in your business clothes.

✔ **Equipment Note:** None required.

Breathing

As you stand aligned, remember to breathe consciously. Observe the breath flowing in and out equally. You may use the Hissing Breath to help you be more conscious of your breathing. Just doing your posture check, Palm Tree Pose, and Hissing Breath exercise (all from Chapter 2) between projects will improve your posture and refresh you.

Stretching

Standing Stretches

These first four stretches are done standing up. However, if you are in a situation where you can't stand up, do the stretches sitting down.

Side Stretch with the Wrist

Stand with your feet hip-width apart and parallel. Check your posture so that you are standing aligned in the Palm Tree Pose. (See Figure 2.8, page 18.)

Inhale and stretch your arms out to the sides and over your head with your palms facing each other. Exhale as you take hold of your left wrist with your right hand.

With an inhalation, stretch the fingers of your left hand to the ceiling. Exhale as you gently stretch to the right, drawing out your left arm and wrist with the right hand and move your hips to the left simultaneously. (See Figure 3.1.) Keep the left arm and head in alignment with the left side of your body. Don't drop your left arm in front of your face. Feel this stretch the entire left side of your body, from your hips to your fingertips.

To keep the feet solidly planted on the floor, press firmly down with your outer left heel. Continue to breathe softly as you stretch to the right, particularly noticing the deep stretch in the left rib cage as the breath enters your left lung.

Inhale as you come back to center. Exhale and switch hands. Holding your right wrist with your left hand, inhale as you reach up through the fingers of your right hand.

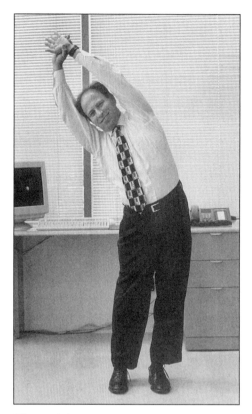

Figure 3.1
Exhale as you stretch to the right, keeping your left arm and head in alignment

Exhale as you stretch to the left. Continue to breathe as you stretch to the left side.

Inhale and return to the center. Repeat this sequence on each side.

✔ **Elise's Note:** This is a great stretch to relieve computer-related tension in your wrists and to stretch your sides. This is a particularly good stretch to relieve lower back tightness.

Chest and Neck Stretch

Interlace your fingers and clasp the back of your head, with your elbows out to the sides. Keep your chin parallel to the floor and lift the crown of your head, feeling a lengthening toward the ceiling.

Inhale, stretch your elbows backwards, and draw your shoulder blades toward each other as you gently arch your back. (See Figure 3.2.) You may feel a stretch in your armpits as your chest expands. This is particularly good if you have a sunken chest.

Exhale and stretch your elbows forward, dropping them toward the floor and pulling the back of your head down with your hands. (See Figure 3.3, page 25.) This movement will lengthen the back of your neck and release tightness in the neck muscles. Feel your jaw, tongue, eye, and face muscles relax as you let the head drop down toward the chest.

Repeat five times.

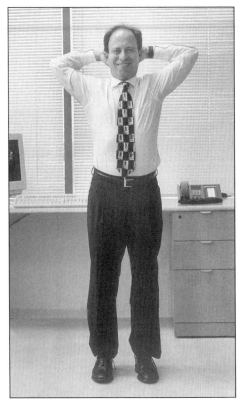

Figure 3.2
As you inhale, stretch your elbows back as you gently arch your back

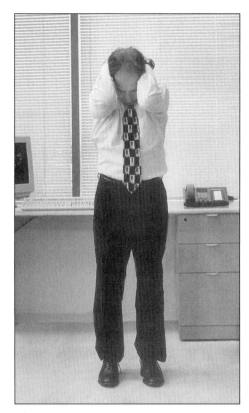

Figure 3.3
As you exhale, bring your elbows
forward as you stretch toward the floor

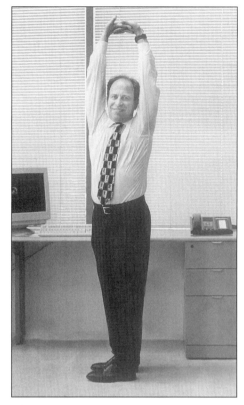

Figure 3.4
Visualize the twist beginning from the
base of your spine

Gentle Twist

Inhale and slowly lift your arms overhead.
Interlace your fingers, stretching the palms
to the ceiling. Be sure to focus on stretching
your wrists, allowing the hands to form
right angles with your forearms.

Exhale and gently twist to the left, keeping
your arms in line with your ears. (See Figure
3.4.) Visualize the twist beginning from the
base of your spine. Feel your navel and chest
revolving to the left. Keep your head in line
with the rest of your body.

Holding your breath while twisting is a
common tendency. Instead, inhale as you
reach up toward the ceiling, and exhale as
you twist a little farther to the left.

When you have twisted as far as your body allows, return to the center on an exhalation. Repeat on the right side.

After your last twist, on an exhalation, bring your arms down by your sides.

This twist helps to bring blood supply to the discs, liver, and kidneys following the "spread, squeeze, and soak" theory that was mentioned in Chapter 1. It also helps to relieve tension in the middle and lower back.

✔ **Elise's Note:** In addition to relieving tension in the middle and lower back, this stretch is also a good way to relieve tension in your wrists.

Mid-Back Stretch

Inhale and slowly lift your arms over your head. Interlace your fingers, stretching your palms to the ceiling. Be sure to focus on stretching your wrists, allowing the hands to form right angles with the forearms.

Exhale and bring your arms to the front, at chest level. Keep your palms facing away from your body.

Inhale, bending your elbows and drawing your hands to your chest. (See Figure 3.5.) At the same time, open and lift your chest toward your hands. Be sure to drop your shoulder blades down toward your waist and drop your elbows down at a forty-five degree angle. Keep your body in alignment, making sure your lower back is in its natural curve.

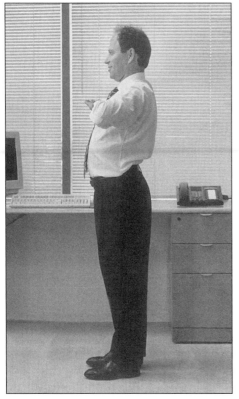

Figure 3.5
As you inhale, draw your hands to your chest while lifting your chest toward your hands

As you exhale, straighten your elbows, pressing your palms away from your chest. (See Figure 3.6.) Round your back and spread your shoulder blades away from your spine. Feel your pelvis tuck and your abdomen move toward your lower back.

Repeat five times.

This stretch relieves tension between the shoulder blades and spine that often happens when you sit at your desk or computer too long.

Sitting Stretches

You may think you know how to sit down. However, many people round their backs, putting stress on the vertebrae of the spine and compressing internal organs. Over time, this can cause back pain and injuries. To sit properly:

Sit on the middle of the chair seat, without leaning on the chair back. Feel your "sitting bones" by placing your hand under each buttock and moving the muscles and flesh to the back. Roll from side to side and you should feel you are sitting on top of your "sitting bones."

Place your hand on your lower back and make sure that there is a slight concave curve. Your spine should be upright and your head and shoulders should be aligned. Lift your head from the base of your skull. (See Figure 3.7, page 28.)

Just reminding yourself to sit in your chair with alignment as you've just done will help with staying alert and help you last longer without getting pain in your back.

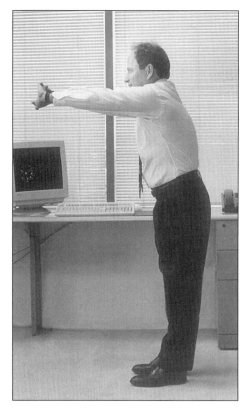

Figure 3.6
As you straighten your elbows, round your back and spread your shoulder blades

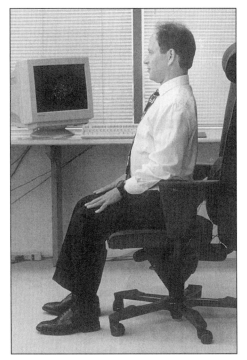

Figure 3.7
To sit properly, sit in the middle of the chair, on your "sitting bones," with your spine straight, and head and shoulders aligned

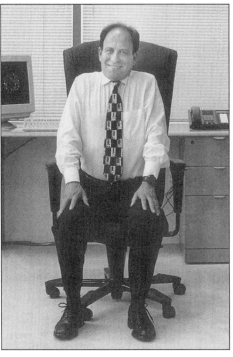

Figure 3.8
Inhale as you lift both shoulders up to your ears

Shoulder Rolls

Sitting upright, inhale as you lift your right shoulder to your ear. Exhale as you slowly roll your shoulder around and back, dropping it away from your ear. Repeat on the other side. Continue these shoulder rolls three more times, alternating right and left.

Now, inhale as you lift both shoulders up to the ears. (See Figure 3.8.) Exhale as you drop them down.

Repeat five times and then relax your shoulders.

Movement is one of the best things you can do for your back if you've been sitting in the same position for a while. This particular movement helps relieve tension in the upper back and shoulders where the trapezius muscle is located.

Upper Body Alignment

Here's an alignment reminder for the upper body. There are three components to this alignment exercise.

Sitting upright, bring your arms out to your sides, with your elbows at right angles slightly above shoulder level.

Part one: Inhale and lift your shoulders up to your ears. Exhale and drop your shoulder blades down toward your waist, focusing on the parts of the shoulder blades that are closest to your spine.

Part two: Keeping your elbows slightly higher than your shoulders, draw your elbows forward and your hands back until you feel your shoulder blades move toward the center of your back. (See Figure 3.9.) You should feel the bottom tip of your shoulder blades pushing forward toward the front of your body. Don't allow your lower ribs to push forward and create a sway back.

Part three: Now push your elbows out against an imaginary force, spreading your shoulder blades away from your spine. Pause and breathe, feeling your uplifted position. Your shoulder blades should be supporting your posture.

Inhale and straighten your elbows, stretching your arms out to your sides with your palms facing up. Turn your thumbs down toward the floor, externally rotating your upper arms. Exhale, keep your uplifted position, and allow your arms to slowly descend.

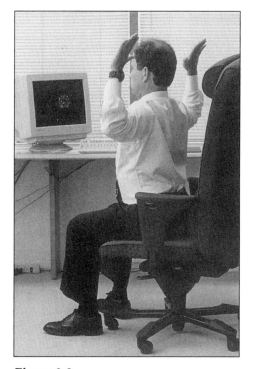

Figure 3.9
Draw your elbows forward and your hands back, feeling your shoulder blades move toward your spine

✔ **Elise's Note:** You may do this standing as well as sitting. What's great about this one is that you can do it anytime, anyplace. One of my students said, "If I didn't learn anything else, this exercise was worth the whole trip. My posture has totally changed." And, in fact, it does change your posture, particularly in the upper back. It also helps to decrease kyphosis, or extreme rounded thoracic spine. This is so powerful because posture is not just about dropping your shoulders away from your ears, it's about dropping your shoulder blades and using them properly to open the chest without pinching between the shoulder blades and the spine. This is using the bone structure of the body rather than overusing the muscles.

Neck Stretch

Sit upright without letting your back touch the back of the chair. Align your head directly over your spine and feel the crown of your head lifting. Hold on to the side of the chair seat with your left hand.

Breathe in, and on exhalation, drop your right ear toward your right shoulder without lifting your right shoulder or turning your head. Take several breaths in and out, feeling the stretch on the left side of your neck.

To create a deeper stretch, reach over your head and place your right hand on the left side of your head to gently pull your neck away from your shoulder. (See Figure 3.10.) At the same time, hold firmly onto the chair with your left hand, and draw your left shoulder away from your neck. Visualize your neck lengthening and the muscles along your vertebrae relaxing. Hold the pose for at least five more breaths.

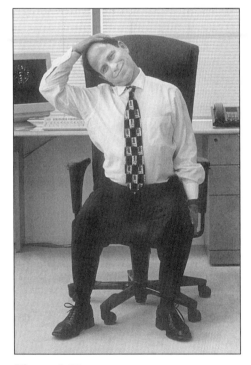

Figure 3.10
For a deeper stretch, gently pull your neck away from your shoulder

You may release your left hand from the chair and gently massage your neck and shoulders with your left hand.

Slowly release and switch sides to repeat the sequence.

This stretch is a great one for a stiff or compressed neck. You can really feel how it lengthens and stretches the neck, creating space between each of the vertebra in the cervical (neck) spine.

Open Chest Stretch

Sit near the edge of a chair and interlace your fingers behind you, with your palms facing your back.

Leaning slightly forward, lift your arms and rest them on the back of the chair. Inhale and lift your chest. Exhale and relax your shoulders away from your ears. (See Figure 3.11.) If your hands do not reach the top of the chair, clasp the sides of the chair back and pull your chest forward, relaxing your shoulders and opening your upper chest.

Hold for ten to fifteen breaths, feeling lightness in your heart.

With an exhalation, slowly release your hands and bring them down by your sides.

As it's named, this one opens the chest, decreasing rounded shoulders and releasing tightness in the mid-back. In addition, it helps decrease kyphosis, or extreme rounded thoracic curve of the back.

✔ **Carol's Note:** After typing at my computer for a long period of time, this one really straightens me out.

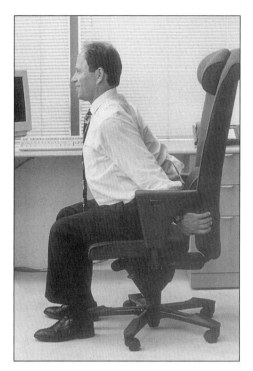

Figure 3.11
Exhale and relax your shoulders away from your ears

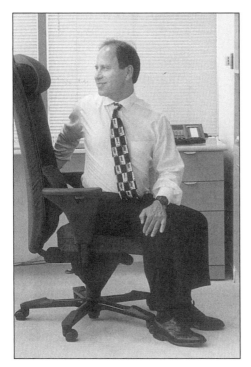

Figure 3.12
Bringing the right arm to the back
of the chair and your left hand on
your right knee, inhale and lengthen
your spine

Chair Twist

Sit toward the front of a chair, then swivel your thighs toward the right side of the chair so you are sitting diagonally on the seat. If you have an arm handle on the side of the chair, bring your thighs as close to it as possible.

Inhale and lift your right arm up to the ceiling. With an exhalation, move your arm to the back of the chair on the opposite side, taking hold of the chair back. Bring the left hand to the right knee or chair handle. Inhale and lengthen your spine. (See Figure 3.12.)

Exhale and twist to the right, pressing your right hand against the back of the chair to deepen the twist. Visualize your shoulder blades dropping down as if they were hanging from weights.

Breathe into your rib cage. Consciously relax the muscles in your back and gently twist a little farther. Stay in the pose for ten to fifteen breaths.

Return to your center with an exhalation and repeat on the opposite side.

Twists are the answer to sitting for long periods of time. After twisting, you will feel the release of all the muscles in your back (particularly in the mid-back) that have been locked into position from sitting a long time. Be sure to do this one all through the day!

Back and Shoulder Release

Part one: Sit on the edge of a chair and place your feet about two and one-half feet apart, parallel to each other. Lean forward and place your forearms on your inner thighs. Press your inner thighs out with your forearms. (See Figure 3.13, page 33.)

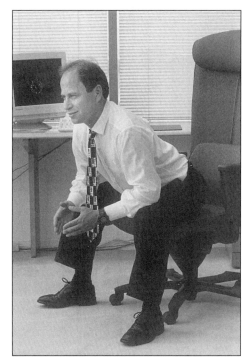

Figure 3.13
Part one: lean forward, pressing your inner thighs out with your forearms

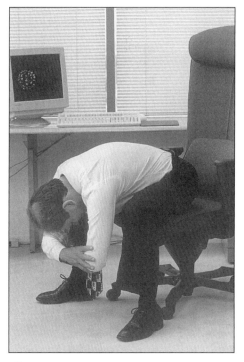

Figure 3.14
Part two: Rest your ribs on your thighs and cross your arms

Breathe deeply in and out, feeling your inner thighs stretching.

Part two: Make sure your knees are directly over your heels and your feet are parallel to each other. Slowly stretch your arms down toward the floor, resting your ribs on your thighs, with your armpits at your knees. Cross your arms, placing your hands at the opposite elbows, releasing downward. (See Figure 3.14.) Continue to breathe deeply.

Part three: For a deeper stretch of the back, stretch your arms forward toward your desk or the floor, reaching through your fingertips and feeling your spine lengthening. (See Figure 3.15.)

Round your back and slowly roll up, returning to a sitting position.

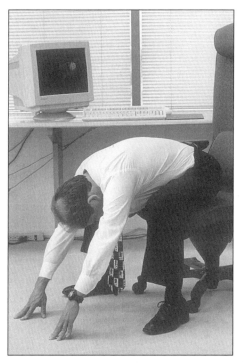

Figure 3.15
Part three: stretch your arms forward, reaching through your fingertips

Relaxation *(Savasana)*

After a stretching session, it is vital to relax deeply to enhance the effectiveness of the poses. Relax sitting up in your chair.

You may record this on audio tape.

Take a slow, deep breath. As you exhale, close your eyes and begin to relax your entire body. Feel your eyes dropping downward toward your cheekbones, letting go of all of your stress.

Begin to feel your neck and shoulders relaxing, all the way down through your arms and into your hands and all the way out into your fingertips.

Begin to observe your breathing. Watch your breath flow in and out like the waves of the ocean. Let your body and mind bathe in the stillness of total relaxation. Take a few minutes to just focus on your breathing, letting everything else drift away.

When you are ready, take a deep breath, open your eyes, and return to your work feeling completely refreshed and alert.

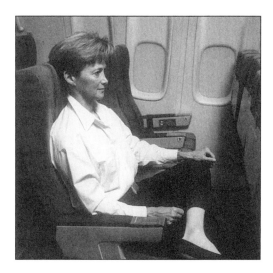

chapter 4

Stretch on a Trip

Do you ever feel . . .

. . . the Wright brothers had more comfortable seats on their airplanes? Your body feels so compressed that you could fold up into your carry-on baggage. The air in the plane is so stale, someone should capture it to study germ cultures from ancient civilizations. You feel exhausted, irritated, and tight in every joint and muscle.

Here are some stretches you can do in your seat or at the back of the airplane cabin. These stretches will bring energy to your body and remind you that you can move all the muscles you used to be able to move back home. One caution: try not to knock out the person beside you. And who knows, maybe you'll start a trend. Two other hints: drink lots of water, and walk around the plane whenever it is possible.

✔ **Equipment Note:** A yoga belt or a belt you are wearing, and an airplane blanket. (If you don't have a belt on you, the airplane blanket will do.)

Breathing

Now that you have settled into your seat and the plane is airborne, it is time to let go of all the stress from preparing for your trip.

Inhale through your nose and exhale through your mouth, letting your jaw drop, and allowing yourself to make the "ahhh" sound, like a relaxing sigh.

Repeat this conscious deep breathing for as many breaths as you need to get settled.

✔ **Carol's Note:** No one will hear you above the sound of the engines. Trust me.

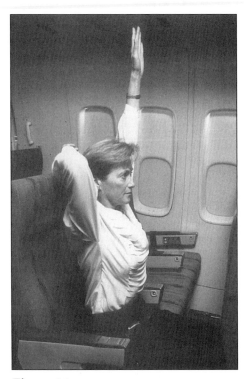

Figure 4.1
Feel the stretch in the mid-back and side, all the way up through your fingers

Stretching

Sitting Stretches

Grapevine Stretches

Inhale and carefully lift your arms over your head (if you touch the ceiling above, bend your elbows), keeping your arms shoulder-width apart. Exhale and relax your shoulders away from your ears.

With an inhalation, stretch the left arm up, reaching with your fingers as if picking fruit from a tree. Keep the right arm relaxed, with the elbow slightly bent. (See Figure 4.1, page 36.) Feel a deep stretch in the muscles between the side ribs as the inhalation expands the chest.

Exhale and relax the left side. Inhale, reaching up with the right arm.

Repeat five times on each side.

You will feel the stretch in the mid-back and side all the way up through the arms to your fingers. This even stretches your ribs and intercostal muscles between the ribs and allows for deeper breathing. Hooray!

Elbow to Ceiling Stretch

Sit in the middle of your seat, stretching up through your spine, with your head in line with your shoulders and pelvis.

Inhale and stretch the right arm up to the ceiling. Exhale and bend the right elbow, bringing your hand to your back. Reach up with your left hand to grasp your right elbow. (See Figure 4.2.)

Pull the elbow back to line up with your right ear. Slide your right hand down your back, stretching your upper arm. Breathe, feeling your shoulder blades moving down toward the front of your body.

With an inhalation, release your left hand from your right elbow. Exhale, stretching your right arm up to the ceiling, and then bring it down to your side.

Repeat twice on each side.

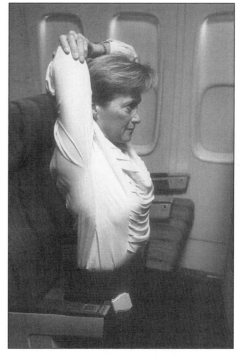

Figure 4.2
As you grasp your right elbow, pull it back, sliding your hand down your back

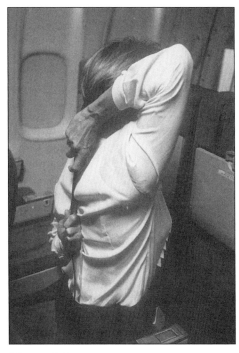

Figure 4.3
If the hands do not reach each other,
use a belt or an airplane blanket

Elbow to Ceiling stretches the upper arm and armpit, opens the chest, and realigns the upper body for better posture.

Shoulder Stretch (*Gomukhasana*)

Sit in the middle of the seat, stretching up through your spine, with your head in line with your shoulders and pelvis.

Inhale, and as you exhale, bend the left elbow behind the back and place the back of the hand on the spine. Slowly move the hand up the back, reaching the fingers toward the neck.

Inhale deeply as you extend the right arm toward the ceiling, and with an exhalation, bend the elbow, stretching the hand down. Clasp the left hand or wrist with the right hand, palms facing each other. If the hands do not reach each other, hold on to both ends of a belt or an airplane blanket. (See Figure 4.3.)

Do not let your head protrude forward. Keep it in line with the rest of the body. As you clasp the hands, visualize the tip of the shoulder blade moving down and in toward the front of the body. At the same time, feel the chest lift.

Hold the pose for ten to fifteen breaths. Repeat on the opposite side.

You will also feel this one stretch the upper arm and armpit and open the chest. It also increases flexibility in the shoulder joint and brings the tips of the shoulder blades in toward the chest, realigning the upper body.

Elbow Stretch

Sit in the middle of your seat, not resting against the back of the seat. Interlace your fingers, keeping your elbows shoulder-width apart.

Inhale, lifting your arms over your head, and lean forward from the hips, placing your forearms on the seat back in front of you. Keep the elbows in line with your shoulders and your fingers relaxed.

Exhale and rest your forehead on the seat back, and push the shoulder blades toward the front of your body. (See Figure 4.4.)

Continue to stay in this position for five breaths, opening the chest and releasing the back.

Slowly inhale, releasing your arms from the back of the seat. Exhale, releasing your fingers and returning your hands to your lap.

✔ **Elise's Note:** You will definitely feel this stretch open the chest and armpits. After I do this one, I'm for sure sitting up a lot straighter!

Shoulder Blade Stretch (*Garudhasana*)

Bend your arms at your elbows to form right angles, with the palms of your hands facing each other.

Inhale as you cross your forearms and grasp the edges of the seat in front of you. (Your right hand should be clasping the left side of the seat, the left hand clasping the right side.) Exhale, rounding your back, and bringing your head forward. (See Figure 4.5.)

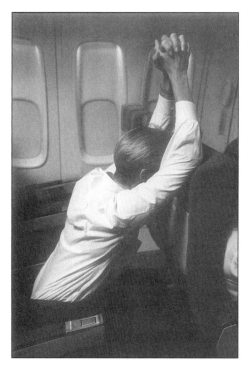

Figure 4.4
Rest your forehead on the seat back as you push the shoulder blades forward

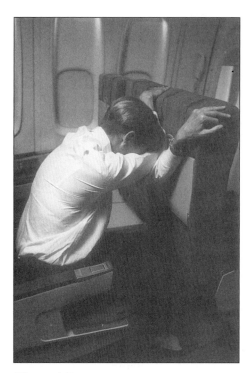

Figure 4.5
Crossing your forearms, grasp the seat in front of you and lean forward

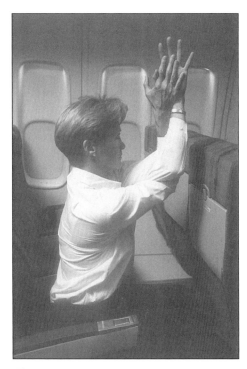

Figure 4.6
A variation of the Shoulder Blade Stretch for those more flexible

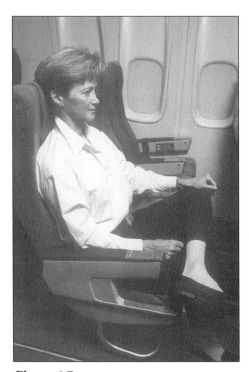

Figure 4.7
Lightly press the knee down, feeling a stretch in the left buttock

Pull your elbows apart. This will spread your shoulder blades, releasing tension between the shoulder blades and the spine. This is where we often feel tension if we sit or hold a position for too long.

Variation

For those of you who are more flexible, bend your arms in front of you, forming right angles with your palms facing.

Cross the left elbow over the right, fitting the left elbow into the notch of the right elbow. Cross your hands and place the fingers of the right hand on the left palm. (See Figure 4.6.)

Breathing in, raise the upper arms to shoulder level, stretching the hands and fingers up. As you slowly exhale, pull the arms away from the body, keeping the hands directly above the elbows without allowing them to move toward the forehead. Visualize the shoulder blades as wings spreading to the sides.

Hold this position for about ten to fifteen breaths, gently breathing into the area between the shoulder blades.

Reverse the arms, bringing the right elbow on top of the left and repeat.

✔ **Carol's Note:** This variation is more challenging. Hang in there.

Hip Opener

Sit with your back straight. For a deeper stretch, sit in the middle of the seat.

Inhale, and with an exhalation, lift your left knee toward your chest.

Interlace your fingers around your shin and draw your leg toward your chest, stretching the mid-back.

Release your hand from your shin and bring your right hand to the bottom of your left foot. Place your left foot on the thigh of your right leg, just above the knee, dropping your left leg.

Exhale and lightly press the knee down with the left hand, feeling a stretch in the left upper leg and buttock. (See Figure 4.7, page 40.)

Hold for ten breaths and repeat on the opposite side.

✔ **Elise's Note:** In addition to these sitting stretches, you can adapt any of the standing and sitting stretches in Chapter 3. Be creative.

Standing Stretches

Wall Stretch

Find a wall in the airplane cabin. Stand facing the wall eighteen inches away, with your feet parallel and hip-width apart.

Inhale and stretch your arms over your head, placing the palms of your hands on the wall, shoulder-width apart. Exhale and bring the forehead to the wall, keeping your hips over your heels. (See Figure 4.8.)

Continue to stretch, walking the hands up the wall, breathing in with one hand and out with other. Feel your upper torso lifting up out of your pelvis.

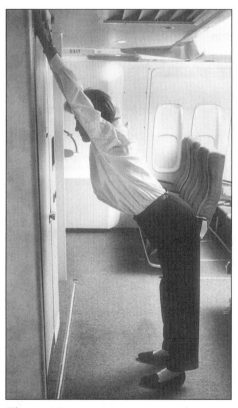

Figure 4.8
Exhale as you bring your forehead to the wall, continuing to stretch as you walk the hands up

Variation

Continuing the Wall Stretch above, if there's room on the plane, slide your hands down so the heels of your hands are in line with the tops of your shoulders. Walk the feet back, keeping them hip-width apart, until you feel a stretch from the heels of the hands through your back all the way to your hips. Make sure the hips are directly over the heels. (See Figure 8.1, page 109.)

Draw the shoulder blades toward the front of the body, feeling the armpits and chest stretching. Align the head with the arms, neither lifting the chin nor dropping it. Exhale and walk the feet back toward the wall, releasing the hands.

You will feel this one in many places depending on where you are tight. Often you will feel it initially in the shoulders and upper body, which will open the chest and improve posture. If you're able to bring the arms down to shoulder level, you will also begin to feel it in the entire back; even the backs of the legs (hamstrings) get a stretch.

Thigh Stretch

Standing eighteen inches away from the wall, feet parallel and hip-width apart, inhale and stretch your arms over your head and place on the wall.

Exhale and bend your left knee, grasping the top of your left foot with your left hand. (See Figure 4.9.)

Stretch down through the left thigh toward the floor, bringing your left knee back and in line with your right leg. Remember to tuck your buttocks so that your tailbone moves toward the front of your body.

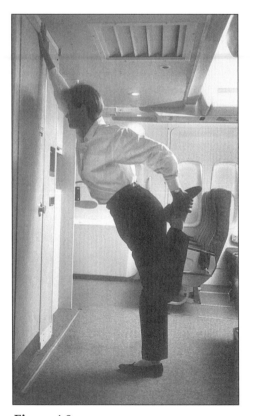

Figure 4.9
Stretch down through your left thigh as you stretch your right arm up the wall

Breathe and stretch your right arm up the wall. Exhale and release your hand from your foot, bringing it back to the floor.

Repeat on the opposite side.

This stretches the front of the thigh, which means you are stretching the quadricep muscle. This muscle needs to be stretched equally with its counter muscle group, the hamstrings, to bring balance to the hip joints and align the pelvis to its normal position.

Shoulder Twist

Stand with the right side of your body six inches away from the wall, with your feet parallel and together.

Inhale and stretch your right arm up the wall, reaching up with your right side all the way through your fingertips.

Exhale and slide your hand down the wall and behind you until your hand is slightly lower than shoulder height. Be sure to drop your shoulder blade down toward your waist while keeping your hand on the wall.

Press your right palm into the wall and bring your right hip forward until it is in alignment with your left hip again. (See Figure 4.10.)

As you exhale, pivot your toes slightly away from the wall and toward your left side, keeping your heels in place. Be sure to align your head with your shoulders, hips, and heels.

Feel the stretch open your chest and your whole upper body as well as bring the right shoulder blade in toward the center of the body. Hold for five breaths.

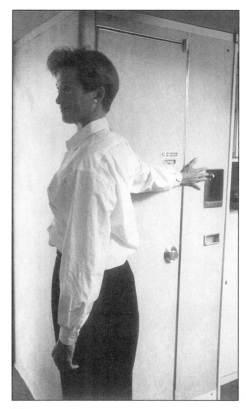

Figure 4.10
Pivot your toes slightly away from the wall, toward your left side, while keeping your head aligned

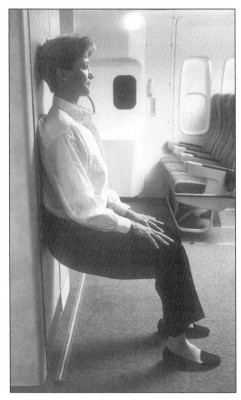

Figure 4.11
Press your lower back into the wall as you hold the position

Exhale and slide your hand down the wall and relax. Repeat on your left side.

✔ **Elise's Note:** During a trip, this helps you realign your body, gives you an uplifted posture, and helps you add more space to take in oxygen and breathe.

Thigh Strengthener

Stand approximately twelve inches away from the wall, with your back to the wall.

Breathe, and with an exhalation, bend your knees until your knees are directly over your ankles. (See Figure 4.11.)

Pause and breathe, feeling your lower back pressing into the wall. Hold for five breaths.

Exhale and press your heels down as you straighten your legs and slide your back up the wall.

This is a thigh burner for sure. It makes those legs good and strong. By strengthening the legs, we bring more support to the spine.

The Squat

Walk the feet back approximately six inches away from the wall.

To come down into a squat, slide the buttocks down the wall, keeping the heels on the floor and not letting the buttocks touch the floor. (See Figure 4.12, page 45.) Keep the pelvis, back, and head at the wall. You may alter the distance from the wall depending on your size.

Stay in the squat, breathing and feeling the stretch in the lower back and buttocks.

Exhale and press your heels down as you straighten your legs and slide your back up the wall.

The squat helps relieve tight muscles in your lower back and buttocks, creating more space between the vertebrae. It's also great for sore buttocks after sitting in the plane for a long time.

If your heels still do not touch the floor, don't despair. Keep stretching through the heels and they eventually will.

Wall Hang *(Uttanasana)*

Stand with your back to a wall, feet hip-width apart and six inches away from the wall. Straighten the knees without locking them back.

Pull up through the shins, knees, and thighs. Clasp your elbows over your head. Inhale and stretch up through your elbows and exhale, bending over from the hips. (See Figure 4.13, page 46.) As you are bending over, reach out and down.

Release your hands and bring them to your buttocks, sliding the buttock muscles up the wall. Place your hands on your elbows again and pull the upper torso down, extending the entire spine. Breathe and hang there for one minute.

Inhale and come up, stretching the elbows out and up. Simultaneously, slide the buttocks down toward the floor, pressing the lower back toward the wall. Exhale and straighten your arms, slowly bringing them down by your sides.

✔ **Elise's Note:** This is a good stretch for the backs of the legs where the hamstring muscle group is located and a wonderful release for the

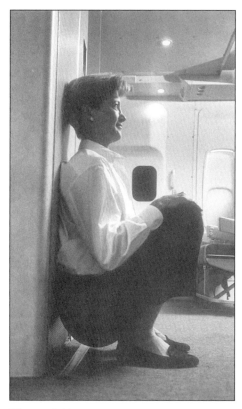

Figure 4.12
As you squat, keep the pelvis, back, and head at the wall

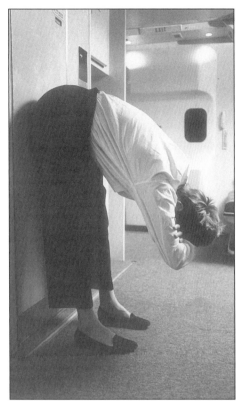

Figure 4.13
As you exhale, bend over from hips, stretching out and down

upper body after sitting on the plane for a long time. If you cannot bend very far, you may use the Wall Stretch. (See Figure 4.8, page 41.)

✔ **Carol's Note:** I like this one. It's the best way I know to practice hanging out.

In addition to these standing stretches, you can adapt any of the standing stretches in Chapter 3.

Relaxation *(Savasana)*

Return to your seat, putting it in a comfortable position, ready to relax. With travel and work stress, the eyes can become strained. Here are some eye exercises to stretch and relax the eyes. We will suggest vertical, horizontal, and circular movements of the eyes. Your reward is a relaxation of the entire body.

You may record this on audio tape.

> Take a deep breath, close the eyes and exhale. Without moving the head, inhale and look up, exhale and look down. Repeat five times.
>
> Without moving your head to the side, inhale and look to the right. Exhale and look to the left. Repeat five times.
>
> Without moving your head, trace the outer rim of a clock by looking up at twelve, going clockwise, moving to three, down to six, around to nine, and up to twelve. Repeat five times clockwise and five times counterclockwise.
>
> Bring the palms of the hands together, rubbing the hands back and forth until they become warm, and cup the palms over the

eyes with the fingertips reaching the hair-line. Breathe in and out, feeling the darkness soothing and relaxing the eyes. Bring the fingertips to the eyelids and gently massage the eyes with circular motions. Keep your eyes closed.

Bring your hands to your lap with the palms facing up. Let your arms and legs completely relax. Feel your back and pelvis sink deeply into your seat. Let all of your senses relax.

Relax your eyes, your ears, your nose, your jaw, and your tongue. Even let the teeth and gums relax. Relax your skull and facial muscles. Remember to observe your breath as you feel your body relax even deeper.

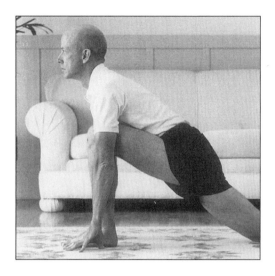

chapter 5

Strengthen and Lengthen Your Lower Back

Do you ever feel . . .

. . . whatever you do, your lower back grips and tightens? You cannot sit at a desk or ride in a car without your back flaring up. You're afraid to do anything new and exciting or you might irritate it. You're trapped in an old body with a young mind and spirit. How do you get your healthy back . . . back?

This chapter features yoga stretches to relieve pain and strengthen your lower back. These stretches give you greater stability and more flexibility. As stated in Chapter 1, yoga alleviates back problems in four ways. It creates movement and flexibility of the back by flexing and extending the spine, thereby generating more blood supply into the discs and preventing and/or healing ruptured discs. Yoga also brings more structural alignment and improves posture, balances the joints and muscles, and re-establishes and maintains the four natural curves of the spine.

To do all this, it is important to strengthen your back in addition to creating more flexibility. Sitting in chairs weakens the back. In order to support the spine, we need to strengthen the muscles as well as release tension. You'll feel strong, relaxed, and able to handle whatever life brings.

✔ **Equipment Note:** A blanket or pillow. Use a yoga sticky mat if you're on a slippery surface, such as a rug, so you don't slide in some of the stretches that require traction.

Breathing

Now that you have finished a busy day, it is time to focus on taking care of your back with a gentle pelvic tilt.

> Lie down on the floor on your back, with your knees bent and your feet placed directly under your knees. Arms are at your sides, with the palms facing up.

> Begin to focus on your breathing by inhaling and tilting your tailbone toward the floor, moving your lower back away from the floor into a concave curve.

Exhale, press the lower back to the floor, lifting the tailbone away from the floor and slightly squeezing the buttocks. Feel the diaphragm move up and relax as the air is released from the lungs.

As you inhale, feel the belly fill with air and the chest expand. Exhale and contract the front of your body while stretching the back.

Repeat ten times.

✔ **Elise's Note:** Not only is this good for breathing, this is a basic back care exercise given to patients by medical doctors, chiropractors, and physical therapists. With this movement, you are flexing and extending the spine with the breath in a gentle rocking motion, which brings blood flow into the discs that it otherwise does not receive. This in turn prevents and heals degenerative disc disease.

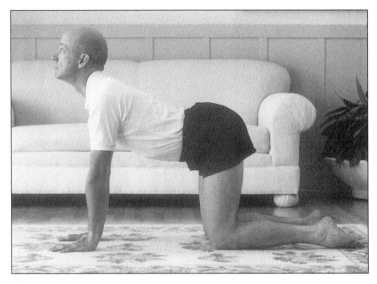

Figure 5.1
Inhale, lifting the head and tailbone while making the lower back concave

Stretching

Cat Cow

Kneel on your hands and knees, with the hands below the shoulders and the knees below the hips. Place a blanket or sticky mat under your knees if you're on a hard surface.

Inhale and lift the head and tailbone, making the lower back concave. (See Figure 5.1.)

Exhale and tuck the tailbone under while rounding the back and releasing the back. (See Figure 5.2, page 53.)

This time as you inhale, feel the fluid movement from the base of your spine to the crown of your head. Drop the shoulders and feel the front of your body stretch.

As you exhale, begin the movement from the pelvis, feeling like you are drawing the navel to the spine, pressing the palms down

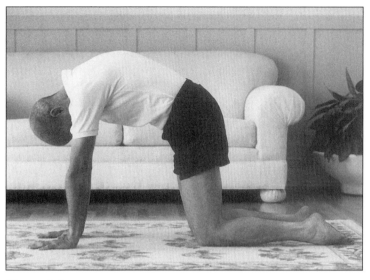

Figure 5.2
Exhale, tucking the tailbone under while rounding the back

into the floor to spread the shoulder blades and lengthen the entire back.

Repeat ten times.

To relax after Cat Cow, it is recommended to go into Child's Pose.

✔ **Elise's Note:** Like the first breathing exercise, the Cat Cow is a pelvic tilt that brings added blood supply and flexibility to the spine, relieves back tension, and prevents degenerative disc disease.

Child's Pose

Kneeling, lay the tops of the feet on the floor. With an exhalation, slowly bring the buttocks back to rest on the heels and bring the arms down to your sides with the palms facing up.

Lower your forehead to rest on the floor and relax the lower back. (See Figure 8.14, page 125.)

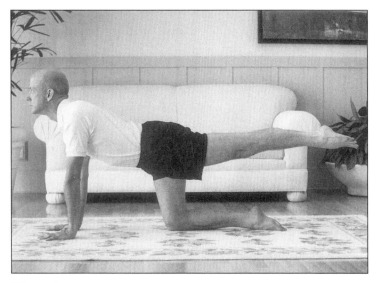

Figure 5.3
Stretch the leg back, pointing the toes and stretching through
the leg

If your buttocks do not reach your heels, use a blanket or pillow to rest on. If your forehead does not touch the floor, use a pillow or blanket to support your forehead.

Breathe and relax for ten breaths.

Remember Child's Pose; it will be used in other stretches in the upcoming chapters.

✔ **Carol's Note:** I like the Cat Cow stretch. It relieves the tension in my entire body, and Child's Pose is my kind of yoga.

Cat Cow with Leg Extension

Kneel on your hands and knees, with the hands below the shoulders and the knees below the hips.

Inhale and stretch the left leg back at hip level, pointing the toes and stretching through the leg. (See Figure 5.3.)

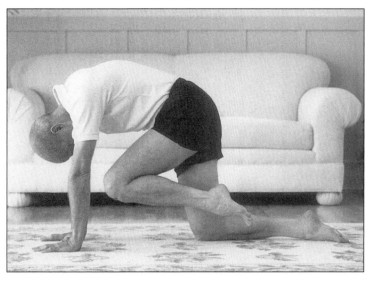

Figure 5.4
Bring the knee to the chest, dropping the forehead toward the knee and rounding the back

Exhale and bring the knee to the chest, dropping the forehead toward the knee and rounding the back. (See Figure 5.4.)

Inhale and stretch the left leg back again, this time stretching through the heel, flexing the toes.

Exhale and bring your knee to your chest, dropping your head.

Continue and repeat four more sets for the left leg, each set including pointing through the toes and stretching through the heel.

Repeat five sets for the right leg, each set including pointing through the toes and stretching through the heel.

When completed, relax into Child's Pose. (See page 53 and Figure 8.14, page 125.)

This stretch not only brings blood supply to the discs when you round and extend your spine, but it also strengthens your back.

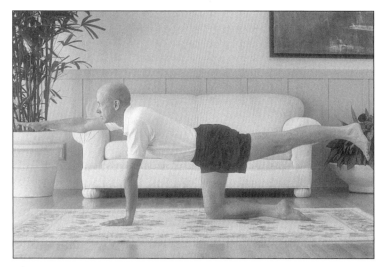

Figure 5.5
For a variation of Cat Cow with Leg Extension (Four-Point Stabilization), extend the leg while stretching the opposite arm out in front

Variation: Four-Point Stabilization

Kneel on your hands and knees, with the hands below the shoulders and the knees below the hips.

Inhale and stretch the left leg back, stretching through the heel and bringing it up to hip level. At the same time, stretch the right arm out in front at shoulder level, stretching from the bottom ribs through the fingertips. (See Figure 5.5.) Pause and breathe.

Exhale and bring the knee and hand back down to the floor.

Repeat with the right heel extended and the left hand stretched out in front. Pause and breathe.

Repeat four times, alternating sides.

If you have trouble with balance, you may want to place the heel of your foot on the wall at hip level.

✔ **Elise's Note:** This stretch is often given by physical therapists to strengthen lower back muscles. You will definitely feel this strengthening your lower back, but if it starts to hurt, come out of it and do Child's Pose. As you do this daily, you will replace tightness with strength!

Extended Puppy Pose (Vajrasana)

To get full benefit from this traction stretch, you will want to be on a non-slippery surface. Use a yoga sticky mat on a rug or simply stretch on the floor with a blanket underneath.

> Kneel on your hands and knees, with the hands below the shoulders and the knees below the hips. Inhale and walk your hands out in front of you.

> Exhale and stretch the buttocks back half-way toward the heels, lengthening the spine. (See Figure 5.6, page 58.) Keep the lower back in its concave curve and press the palms to the floor, keeping the arms off the floor. Feel the arms and the pelvis stretching away from each other, with the upper back following the arms and the lower back following the pelvis. Allow the forehead to relax on the floor.

> Breathe into this position, feeling the muscles between the ribs stretching and the spine and back muscles lengthening. Take fifteen breaths in this posture.

> To release out of this pose, slowly move the buttocks all the way back to the heels and relax the arms by your sides into Child's Pose. (See page 53 and Figure 8.14, page 125.) Totally relax.

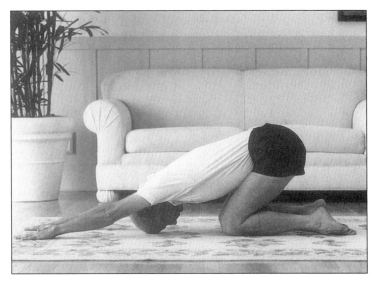

Figure 5.6
Exhale and stretch the buttocks back halfway toward the heels, lengthening the spine

✔ **Elise's Note:** This stretch creates more space between the vertebrae of the spine, thereby reducing compression of nerves and tightness of muscles. You may want to have your side next to a mirror to make sure your lower back remains concave (inward). This is important to feel the pose deeply.

✔ **Carol's Note:** This is another one of my favorites. Feel the stretch in your back and buttocks. Just let all of your tension go away.

Kneeling Lunge

Kneel on your hands and knees, with the hands below the shoulders and the knees below the hips.

Inhale and bring the left foot forward, placing the foot between the hands.

Exhale and lunge the left knee forward, bringing the knee slightly in front of the

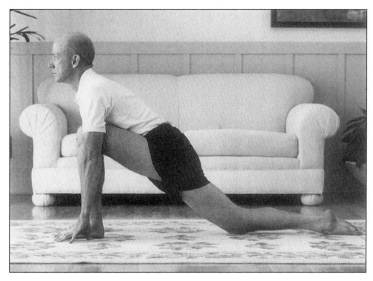

Figure 5.7
Exhale and lunge the left knee forward, lowering the right thigh down to the floor

ankle bone, lowering the right thigh down to the floor. (See Figure 5.7.) This stretches the front thigh muscle (quadricep) and psoas muscle.

Stay in the pose for ten breaths. Repeat on opposite side.

To deepen the stretch, bring the hands to the thigh. Push the palms into the thigh as you lunge deeper.

✔ **Elise's Note:** This stretches the front thigh muscle group (quadriceps) and psoas muscle. The iliopsoas, commonly known as the psoas (sō´ăz) muscle, is very important to stretch. This muscle runs along both sides of your body from the inner thigh bones diagonally from front to back, attaching to the lower back. (See Figure 5.8.) In addition to flexing your thigh to your chest, the psoas muscle affects your posture. When it becomes tight, your torso is thrust forward and you are out of alignment, creating tension and causing pain in the lower back.

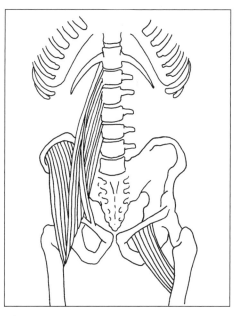

Figure 5.8
Illustration of the psoas muscle

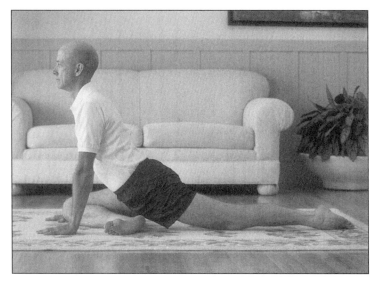

Figure 5.9
Be sure your foot is placed as far forward as possible, using your hand to guide your heel to point to your hip

Hip Opener

Kneel on your hands and knees, with the hands below the shoulders and the knees below the hips.

Slide the right knee forward, bringing the right foot in front of the left thigh. (See Figure 5.9.) Make sure your right foot is placed as far forward as possible, using your hand to guide your heel to point to your left hip. Keep your weight centered and your hips parallel, so that the left hip is not higher than the right.

Inhale, lifting up through the spine. Exhale, sliding your upper body forward, bringing your forearms on to the floor. (See Figure 5.10, page 61.)

Stay in the pose for at least one minute, remembering to breathe.

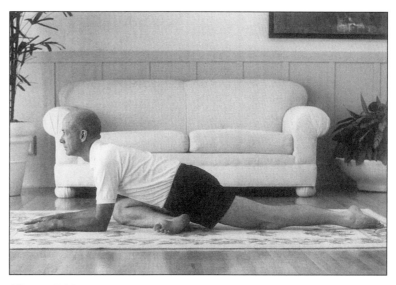

Figure 5.10
Exhale while sliding your upper body forward to bring your forearms to the floor

Slowly inhale and come back up on your hands. Exhale and slide the right leg back so that you are again on your hands and knees.

Repeat on the opposite side.

If you are more flexible, you may stretch the arms all the way out in front of you and bring your forehead to the floor. If you are less flexible and cannot bring your forearms to the floor, keep the hips level and gradually walk your hands out toward the front.

✔ **Elise's Note:** This stretches the buttock muscles, including the piriformis muscle near where the sciatic nerve runs. Although this is not a classic yoga pose, it is a wonderful stretch for anyone suffering from sciatica or nerve compression, which often creates pain or numbness down the legs.

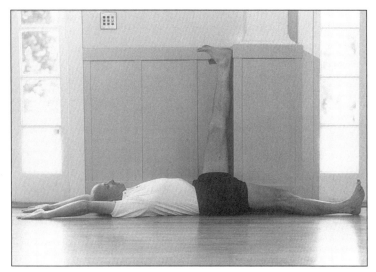

Figure 5.11
With the left leg on the wall, stretch up through the heel, flexing the toes, trying to straighten the knee

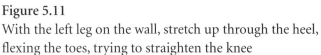

Hamstring Stretch on a Corner **(Supta Padangusthasana)**

Find a doorway or a partial wall and lie down, with your left side next to it. Raise your left leg up on the doorway or wall, so that your left buttock is up against it. Extend your right leg on the floor, with the right inner thigh next to the edge of the doorway or wall. (See Figure 5.11.)

If your chin is higher than your forehead, place a blanket under your head to lengthen the back of your neck.

Stretch up through the left heel, flexing the toes toward the shin, feeling your hamstring muscle in the back of your leg stretch. Your goal is to straighten your knee because your hamstring attaches from below your knee to your buttocks. Also stretch through the right heel, flexing the toes.

Press the right thigh down to the floor. Stay in this pose for a minimum of one minute.

Repeat on the opposite side.

Don't forget to breathe and try not to make such a face. Remember, it takes fewer muscles to smile than frown!

If you do not feel a stretch in this pose, you may place a belt on the ball of your left foot and pull your leg toward your chest, keeping the knee straight. If your hamstrings and lower back are extremely tight, bend the right knee and place your right foot on the floor. Maintain the natural curve in your lower back as you stretch up through the heel.

✔ **Elise's Note:** As you may have guessed or felt by now, this stretches the hamstrings located in the back of your upper leg. The reason this muscle is so important to stretch for lower back problems is that it attaches up in the buttocks and if the hamstrings are tight it will in turn tighten the lower back and pelvic area. This can even create a less than normal natural concave (inward) curve in the lower back, creating bad posture and back problems. You can really see progress in your hamstrings releasing by staying in this pose for a while. This is a real "hang loose" pose so stay with it!

✔ **Carol's Note:** Even grab a magazine or a newspaper, or for the dedicated, grab your favorite novel.

Back Strengtheners

Remember that these are important for maintaining posture, stability of the spine, and balance of muscles and joints.

Staff or Rod Pose (*Dandasana*)

Sit on the floor with your legs together in front of you. Make sure you're sitting on the bottom bones of your pelvis known as the "sitting bones." Place a hand under one buttock and roll the skin out to the side, getting the muscles out of the way to feel the bones. Do the same with the opposite side.

Stretch through your heels, pressing your thighs to the floor. (See Figure 8.9, page 119.) Lift the arms out to the side and overhead. See if you can bring the lower back into its natural curve and lift the arms from the lower back rather than just from the shoulder sockets.

Breathe and feel the stretch as well as the strengthening of the muscles. After ten breaths, slowly bring the arms down by your sides.

Seems deceivingly simple but what an effort! If you could hardly do this and keep the lift and your natural curves, you are a candidate for the following back strengtheners. That includes all of us. So coming up are three variations of back strengtheners.

Back Strengthener Variation One

Lie flat on your abdomen, with your arms stretched out in front.

Inhale and stretch your right arm out. Exhale and stretch your left arm out.

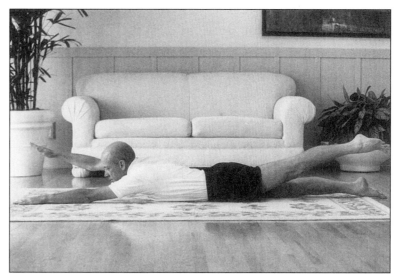

Figure 5.12
Lift your right arm up as you squeeze the left buttock and lift your left leg up, stretching through the toes

Continue to walk the hands out in front with your breathing, until you feel a stretch in your whole upper body.

Press your left palm down. Inhale and lift your right arm up. Squeezing the left buttock, exhale and lift your left leg up, stretching through the toes. (See Figure 5.12.) Keep an equal height of the right arm and left leg. Be sure your head is in line with your spine, not lifting the chin or dropping the head.

Breathe and stretch your arm and leg away from each other. Hold for five breaths. Exhale and release.

Repeat, bringing your left arm and right leg up.

When finished, relax by placing the left side of your head on the floor and closing your eyes. Feel the back relax.

This stretches and strengthens the back at the same time.

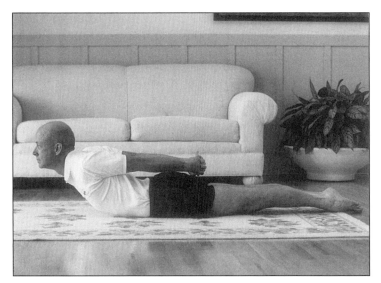

Figure 5.13
Exhale and lift the upper torso, stretching the arms back,
squeezing the shoulder blades together

Back Strengthener Variation Two

Lie flat on your stomach and interlace your fingers behind your back, with the palms facing toward your head. Elbows are extended and your fingers are at the buttocks.

Inhale and squeeze the buttocks. Exhale and lift the upper torso, stretching the arms back, squeezing the shoulder blades together, and lifting the hands toward the ceiling. (See Figure 5.13.) Keep your head in line with your spine, not lifting the chin or dropping the head.

Pause and take three breaths.

On an exhalation, lift both legs from the floor, stretching through the toes. Pause and take three breaths.

Exhale and release, slowly bringing the arms and legs down to the floor.

When finished, relax by placing your right cheek on the floor and closing your eyes. Feel the back relax.

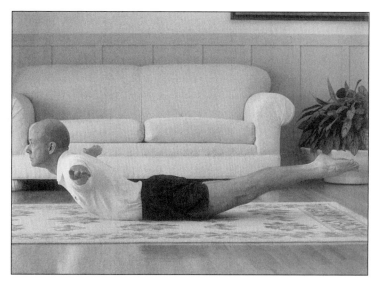

Figure 5.14
Squeeze the buttocks and lift the arms and legs simultaneously

This second variation draws the shoulder blades in toward each other and also toward the front of the body. You may feel this open the chest and decrease rounding in the mid-back (kyphosis).

Back Strengthener Variation Three

Lie flat on your abdomen and slide the arms out to your sides, in line with the top of your shoulders.

Breathe as you stretch out through your fingers, stretching your shoulder blades away from your spine.

Inhale and squeeze the buttocks. Exhale and lift the arms and legs simultaneously. (See Figure 5.14.) Be sure your head is in line with your spine, not lifting the chin or dropping the head. Continue to stretch your shoulder blades away from your spine.

Pause and take six breaths.

Exhale and release the arms and legs down to the floor.

When finished, relax by placing the left side of your head on the floor and closing your eyes. Feel the back relax.

This last variation spreads the shoulder blades and creates more space across the back as well as strengthening the back.

Crocodile Twist

Lie flat on your back. Place a blanket under your head if your chin is higher than your forehead.

Stretch your arms out to your sides, in line with the tops of your shoulders. Open the palms to the ceiling and press the tops of your shoulders into the floor.

Bend both knees, feet flat on the floor. Lift the buttocks. Move and place the hips on the floor to the left so that they are in line with the left shoulder.

Inhale and bring the right leg down to the floor, stretching through your heel. Exhale and place the left foot on top of the right thigh, knee facing toward the ceiling.

Inhale and stretch out through the fingers of the left hand. Exhale and roll on to the right hip, twisting to the right and bringing your right thigh down toward the floor. (See Figure 5.15, page 69.)

Turn your head to the left. Be sure to keep the left shoulder on the floor as you extend through your right heel.

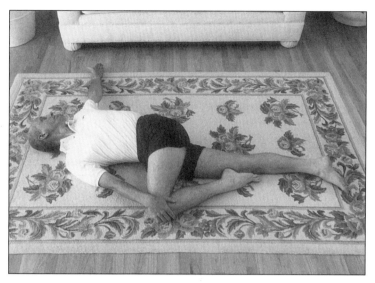

Figure 5.15
Exhale and roll on to the right hip, twisting to the right and bringing your right thigh down toward the floor

Hold for five breaths.

To deepen the stretch, place your right hand on your left thigh. On an exhalation, stretch your knee toward the floor without lifting your left shoulder from the floor.

✔ **Carol's Note:** Congratulations on completing this one without tying yourself in a knot. Actually, this feels great.

If you want more stretching for your hips and hamstrings, check out Chapter 8 on stretching for sports.

Relaxation *(Savasana)*

You may record this on audio tape.

Lie flat on your back on the floor, with your legs straight out in front. You can get a pillow or blanket to put under your knees so that your lower back can totally relax. If you still feel tension, place your calves on the seat of a chair.

Bring the right knee toward the chest and interlace your fingers around your shin, gently hugging your leg, and visualize breathing into your lower back. Repeat on the left side.

Stretch your legs back out to the starting position and rest your arms at your side.

Relax the whole body, letting the arms and legs sink into the floor. Be sure to let the inner thighs, the lower legs, and the toes roll away from the body in a natural position. Make sure your head is aligned and your eyes are closed and relaxed.

Relax all of the muscles in your face and let go of all thoughts. Focus on your breathing and visualize the breath moving down into the lower back and pelvic area.

Inhale and squeeze your buttock muscles. Exhale and totally let the buttock muscles, lower back, and belly relax. Feel all of the organs in the lower pelvic region let go.

As you exhale, feel the diaphragm relax, allowing the lower back to soften into the floor. Feel your body relax even deeper.

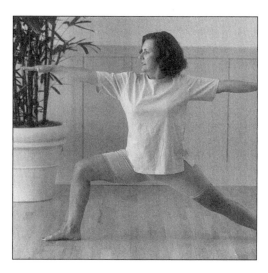

chapter 6

Change Fat to Firm in Thighs and Legs

Do you ever feel . . .

. . . aerobic exercise can be good for you, but you are not exactly breaking attendance records? The ripples in your thighs continue to multiply by the minute. You have considered the possibility that cellulite might be taking over your entire body. Your knees and back ache every time you try to keep up with the hard-bodied types who must secretly live at the gym. Now fight back with your own secret weapon.

Here's how to change fat to firm with some safe and solid yoga stretches that strengthen the thighs and legs. Sounds like a contradiction, doesn't it: "stretches that strengthen"? Actually, not at all. Yoga has the beauty of stretching one muscle group while strengthening another.

In this chapter, you will be asked to hold the poses, ideally, for one minute. To judge the time, count the number of breaths you take in one minute. In the beginning you will want to hold these poses for fifteen to thirty seconds until you build up strength, so also calculate how many breaths that is. Then consistently use that number of breaths to judge your time. Set your timer and try this now.

✔ **Equipment Note:** A yoga sticky mat (if you're on a slippery surface or a rug), a chair, a yoga block or a book, a blanket, and a kitchen timer or watch.

Breathing

To prepare to exercise, stand barefoot on a floor without a rug if possible. With your feet together, toes and heels touching, feel your heels descend down into the floor as if they are roots stabilizing you. Check your posture by doing Palm Tree Pose. (See Figure 2.8, page 18.)

Lift the toes and feel the ankles and front thighs lift up. Squeeze and lift the thighs right above the knees, feeling the lift. This will prevent you from locking your knees and overstretching the backs of your knees, yet keeping the legs straight.

Inhale and exhale, gently spreading the toes, creating space between each toe.

Gently bring the toes down to the floor without the ankles or thighs dropping. Be sure that your hips are directly over your ankles, placing the pelvis in a "neutral" position. Neutral means that the top of your pelvis is parallel to the floor, neither tucking your buttocks nor pushing the tailbone back.

Inhale and lift the shoulders and exhale, dropping the shoulders down toward the waist. Notice your chest open. Align your head, shoulders, pelvis, and ankles. Keeping the upper body relaxed, feel the strength in your legs. Breathe in and out, noticing your alignment.

Stretching

Knee Lift

Place your back against the wall, with your feet four inches away and parallel, hip-width apart. Place your palms against the wall by your sides and inhale.

Exhale and begin to lift the right leg, stretching through your heel, flexing the toes back toward the shin. Keep the head and shoulders at the wall. (See Figure 6.1.)

Press your palms to the wall to lift your leg higher. With the leg unsupported, this is a thigh strengthener in addition to being a gentle hamstring stretch.

Breathe and hold for ten to fifteen seconds, increasing your time as you practice.

Exhale, bringing the leg down to the floor.

Repeat twice on each side.

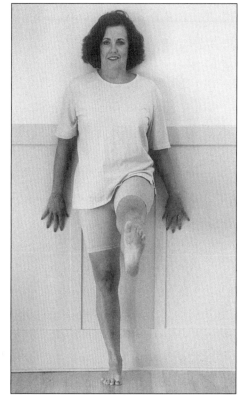

Figure 6.1
Lift the left leg, stretching through the heel, flexing the toes toward the shin

✔ **Elise's Note:** This stretch teaches you to lift your kneecap and contract the quadriceps, which is often required in many of the following standing poses. This stretch is often given to patients who need therapy after knee surgery to strengthen the thigh.

Tree Pose (Vrksasana)

Stand in Palm Tree Pose. (See Figure 2.8, page 18.) Feel your weight equally distributed between your feet.

Inhale and on exhalation, shift your weight to your right foot and lift your left heel to your right thigh. Press the left heel into the inner thigh and the thigh into the heel, creating an equal pressure.

Bring the hands to the hips, making sure your hips are level. Stretch out through the left thigh. Firm the left buttock and begin to bring the left knee back in line with the right hip. Be sure to keep the right hip from coming forward.

Place the palms together at chest level. (See Figure 6.2.) Breathe and maintain your balance. The position of the palms is a greeting position often practiced in India, known as *Namaste*.

When you can balance with your hands at your chest, bring the arms down by your sides, palms facing up.

Inhale and stretch your arms over your head, palms facing each other. Lift up through the spine and breathe. (See Figure 6.3, page 75.)

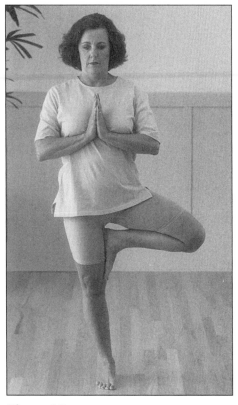

Figure 6.2
Bring the bent knee back in line with the hips

If you can, hold this pose for one minute, or do it twice for half a minute each time in the beginning.

Inhale, and on an exhalation, bring the right foot down to the floor. Return to Palm Tree Pose.

Repeat on the opposite side.

✔ **Elise's Note:** This pose is good for strengthening the legs and opening the inner thighs as well as balancing the body and the mind. You feel more centered and focused practicing this pose.

✔ **Carol's Note:** If you find yourself falling over, don't worry. Place your back against a wall and learn to balance that way first.

Zig Zag Pose (Utkatasana)

Stand in Palm Tree Pose. (See Figure 2.8, page 18.) Inhale and stretch your arms over your head with your palms facing.

Join the palms, crossing the thumbs, and stretch up through the spine and forefingers with your upper arms touching the backs of your ears. If your elbows bend, keep your hands shoulder-width apart and stretch up through your fingers to the ceiling. Breathe, feeling the lift of the chest all the way from your pelvis.

Keeping the heels down and the arms and upper torso lifted, bend the knees a third of the way down toward the floor. (See Figure 6.4, page 76.) Keep lengthening the lower back toward the tailbone and stretching the lower ribs toward the ceiling. Keep the shoulder blades pulling in toward the chest and stretch the abdomen. Also stretch the front and back ribs up evenly to the ceiling.

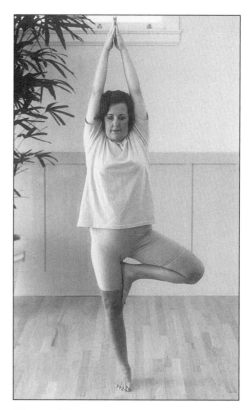

Figure 6.3
Stretch your arms overhead, lifting up through the spine

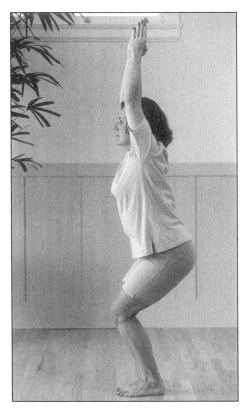

Figure 6.4
As you bend, lengthen the back, stretch the lower ribs, shoulder blades, and abdomen

Breathe and hold for thirty seconds at first, building up to one minute.

With an exhalation, press down through the heels, straighten the legs, and bring the arms down to your sides.

✔ **Elise's Note:** This is one of the best poses for strengthening the legs, and it gives your spine a lift at the same time.

Triangle Pose (Trikonasana)

This is a classic yoga pose. You may find this pose a bit more complex, so be patient when first trying this one.

Stand in Palm Tree Pose. (See Figure 2.8, page 18.) Place your feet four feet apart, with your toes facing forward. Stretch the arms to the sides at shoulder level. Straighten the knees without locking them.

Pull up through the shins, knees, and thighs. Turn the left foot slightly in toward the center of the body. Turn the right leg ninety degrees to the right with the right heel in line with the instep of the left foot. Feel your thighs rolling away from each other so that the right knee is over the right foot and the left knee faces forward.

Exhale and bend sideways toward the right leg, placing the right palm on the lower leg, forming a triangle.

Extend the left arm up to the ceiling, palm facing forward. (See Figure 6.5, page 77.) Be sure to keep your head, shoulders, and left arm in line with your right leg.

As the upper body bends to the right, be sure to move your hips to the left.

Allow your head to look up toward your left hand. If your neck is tense, keep your head facing forward.

Breathe and hold for one minute.

Inhale and press down with the outer left heel and come up. Return to the center.

Repeat on the left side. At the end of the second side, bring the feet back together in Palm Tree Pose.

✔ **Elise's Note:** This pose covers all the bases. It stretches the hamstrings, opens the hips and chest, and aligns the whole body.

✔ **Carol's Note:** This is yoga's answer to the "rack." If you can do this one, you are close to perfection.

Warrior II (**Virabhadrasana II**)

Stand in Palm Tree Pose. (See Figure 2.8, page 18.) Place your feet four and one-half to five feet apart, with your toes facing forward. Stretch the arms to the sides at shoulder level. Straighten the knees without locking them.

Pull up through the shins, knees, and thighs. Turn the left foot slightly in toward the center of the body. Turn the right leg ninety degrees to the right with the right heel in line with the instep of the left foot. Feel your thighs rolling away from each other so that the right knee is over the right foot and the left knee faces forward.

Exhale and bend the right leg so that your right knee is over the right heel and your thigh is parallel to the floor, creating a right angle to the floor as if sitting in a chair. (See Figure 6.6, page 78.)

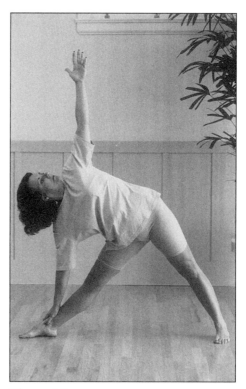

Figure 6.5
As you extend, keep your head, shoulders, and arm in line with your right leg

Change Fat to Firm in Thighs and Legs • 77

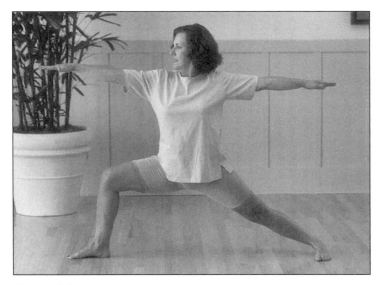

Figure 6.6
As you bend, the right knee should be over the right heel with the thigh parallel to the floor

Turn your head to the right, looking over your right arm. Drop your shoulders away from your ears. Be sure to keep your upper body centered between your legs.

Press the left outer heel down to the floor, keeping the left leg firm. Pull the right knee toward the right side so that it lines up over your right outer heel, and tuck your tailbone in. Feel equal weight on both legs. If you feel your body leaning toward the front leg, imagine someone pulling you back through your left wrist until you feel a slight crease in your left hip.

Breathe and hold for thirty seconds at first, building up to one minute.

Inhale and press down with the outer left heel, straighten the right leg and come up.

Return to the center and repeat on the opposite side.

✔ **Elise's Note:** You may not be able to come down to the right angle in the beginning. As your inner thighs release and your legs become stronger, you will be able to form a right angle. The important alignment is to keep your right knee over your right heel. If your knee is over your toes, walk your left foot back farther. This is also great for strengthening the legs and feeling centered. I call this one the "peaceful warrior."

Right-Angled Side Stretch (Utthita Parsvakonasana)

This is another more complex classic yoga pose.

Stand in Palm Tree Pose. (See Figure 2.8, page 18.) Place your feet four and one-half to five feet apart, with your toes facing forward, and stretch the arms to the sides at shoulder level. Straighten the knees without locking.

Pull up through the shins, knees, and thighs. Turn the left foot slightly in toward the center of the body. Turn the right leg ninety degrees to the right with the right heel in line with the instep of the left foot. Roll your thighs away from each other so that the right knee is over the right foot and the left knee faces forward.

Exhale and bend the right leg so that your right knee is over the right heel and your thigh is parallel to the floor, creating a right angle to the floor. Inhale and press the left outer heel into the floor.

Exhale, extending the right side of the body out, and reach out and down with your right hand, placing your hand on the little-toe side of your right foot. Be sure that your knee presses against your upper arm.

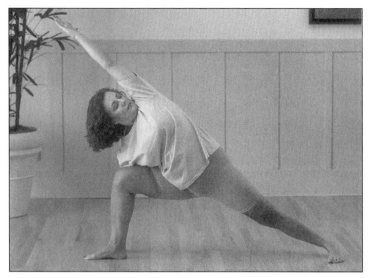

Figure 6.7
Be sure you have created a diagonal line from your heel
through the outstretched fingertips

Place your left hand at your waist. Inhale,
squeezing the buttocks, and exhale, drawing your left shoulder back to open your
chest. Align your body so you are not facing the floor.

Bring your left arm down toward your left
thigh, with your palm facing the ceiling.
Inhale, pressing your outer left heel to the
floor, and exhale, stretching your arm over
your head, bringing it next to your left ear.
(See Figure 6.7.)

Look up at your left arm. Make sure you
have created a diagonal line from your
outer left heel through the fingertips of
your left hand.

Breathe and hold for thirty seconds at first,
building up to one minute.

Inhale and press down with the outer left
heel, straighten the upper body and the
right leg, and come up.

Return to center and repeat on the opposite side.

If you cannot reach the floor, you may grab your ankle or place a book or a yoga block on the floor next to your foot to rest your hand. If that is too difficult, place your right forearm on your right thigh and bend only as far as you can.

✔ **Elise's Note:** Although this stretch may be difficult for you, you will feel it strengthen the legs, stretch the inner thighs, open the upper torso, and stretch the sides of your body.

✔ **Carol's Note:** This is the "rack" revisited. Hang in there.

Standing Forward Bend (**Uttanasana**)

Stand in Palm Tree Pose. (See Figure 2.8, page 18.) Your feet are hip-width apart. Bring your hands to the crease where your legs meet your torso, placing your forefingers in front and your thumbs at your sides.

Inhale, lift up through your spine. Exhale and bend over at your hips, dropping your upper body toward the floor. Be sure to keep your thighs lifted and knees straight.

Slowly release your hands and clasp your elbows, stretching down through the sides of your body. (See Figure 6.8.) Release your neck and head.

Breathe and hold for thirty seconds.

Bring your hands back to the tops of your legs. Inhale and extend your spine as you come up halfway, with your upper body parallel to the floor.

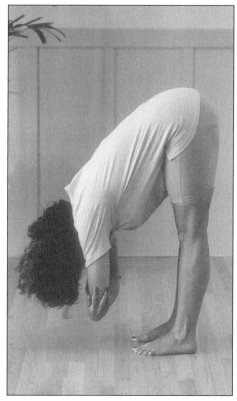

Figure 6.8
Stretch down through the sides of your body, releasing your neck and head

To lift the upper body completely to a vertical position, press down through your heels, lifting through your thighs, feeling the support through your legs, and slowly come up tucking your buttocks.

Variation

If your hands can reach the floor, place your fingers on the outsides of your feet in line with your toes. If you can't quite reach, you may place a block in front of your feet and place your hands on the block. Bring some weight forward into the balls of your feet and your fingers. Be sure that your hips and ankles are in line.

Release your abdomen, neck, and head. Breathe and hold for thirty seconds.

Bring your hands back to the tops of your legs. Inhale and extend your spine as you come up halfway, with your upper body parallel to the floor.

To lift the upper body completely to a vertical position, press down through your heels, lifting thorough your thighs, feeling the support through your legs.

✔ **Elise's Note:** This is the ultimate hamstring stretch. If your hamstrings are extremely tight and you're rounding your back from the waist, do the Right-Angled Wall Stretch. (See Figure 8.1, page 109.) An important part of this posture is coming back up. This is the best training to learn to use your legs to lift your back out of a forward bend correctly.

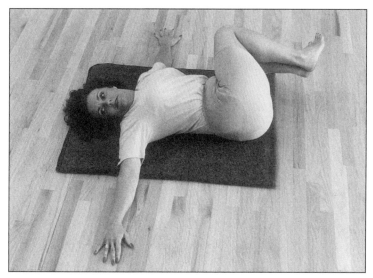

Figure 6.9
Exhale and twist your knees to the left, keeping your right shoulder down and your knees off the floor, turning your head to the right

Floor Twist (Jathara Parivartanasana)

Lie down on your back, with your knees bent and your feet flat on the floor, hip-width apart. Place a blanket under your head if your chin is higher than your forehead.

Move your arms out to the sides, in line with the tops of the shoulders, palms facing down. Move and place the hips to the right so that they are in line with the right shoulder.

Exhale and pull the knees up to your chest. Inhale and stretch through your heels, and flex the toes toward the shins. Keep your knees, big toes, and heels together.

Exhale and twist your knees to the left, keeping your right shoulder down and your knees off the floor. Turn your head to the right. Breathe and hold for one minute. (See Figure 6.9.)

To deepen the stretch, place your left hand on your right thigh and stretch your knee toward the floor. Move your right knee forward to line up with your left knee without lifting your right shoulder off the floor. Keep extending through your heels, keeping your feet from touching the floor.

Exhale and return your knees to the center and place your feet flat on the floor. Lift your hips back to the center.

Repeat on the opposite side, moving and placing your hips to the left to twist to the right.

✔ **Elise's Note:** If you feel a strain in your back or your legs are tired, let the feet and thighs drop to the floor in this pose. You will feel this twist in the mid-back and lower back. This helps back stiffness and brings better circulation to your abdomen and waist.

Bridge Pose (Setu Bandha Sarvangasana)

Lie down on your back, with your knees bent and your feet flat on the floor, hip-width apart. Move your arms down by your sides, with your palms facing down.

Inhale and press the palms down. Exhale and press the heels into the floor, squeezing the buttocks and lifting the pelvis up toward the ceiling. (See Figure 6.10, page 85.)

Interlace your fingers under your buttocks, extending through the elbows to keep your arms straight. Keep your knees parallel and press your inner thighs toward each other.

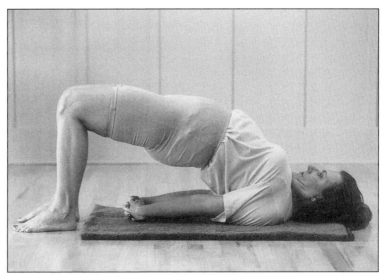

Figure 6.10
Exhale and press the heels into the floor, squeezing the buttocks and lifting the pelvis up

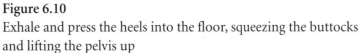

Breathe and hold for thirty seconds, building up to one minute.

Release the fingers, stretch the arms over the head. Exhale and slowly bring your spine down to the floor, vertebra by vertebra, lengthening the pelvis toward your heels.

Repeat this sequence.

Variation

To come up higher on the tops of your shoulders, shift your weight onto the right shoulder and roll the left shoulder around and under, bringing it toward the center of the body, so that you may rest on the top of your left shoulder. Now shift your weight to your left shoulder and roll your right shoulder around and under. Equalize your weight on both shoulders. Press your heels and little fingers into the floor as you feel your chest move toward your chin.

To lift your pelvis up higher, lift the heels, pressing the balls of the feet into the floor. If you can reach, you may also place your hands at your waist, with elbows on the floor, to support your lower back.

✔ **Elise's Note:** This is a pose that strengthens the back and hamstrings and at the same time stretches the quadriceps and psoas muscle. You will also feel it opening your chest to help you breathe deeper. Since we tend to round our shoulders forward, it also helps us realign our bodies into a more open posture. It relieves tightness in the thoracic spine and decreases kyphosis. Many doctors and chiropractors recommend this exercise for therapeutic back care.

Relaxation *(Savasana)*

You may record this on audio tape.

Lie flat on your back on the floor. Align your head with the center of your body. Bring your hands to your head and place your thumbs at the base of your skull. To lengthen your neck, press your thumbs into your skull and move your head away from your neck. If your chin is still higher than your forehead, place a blanket under your head.

Bring your arms down by your sides, forty-five degrees away from your thighs to allow your shoulders to drop down to the floor. Be sure that your shoulders are dropped away from your ears.

Let your back and pelvis sink into the floor. Bring your awareness to your right leg. Slowly lift your right leg two inches from the floor. Inhale and squeeze all of the muscles in your right leg. Exhale and drop the leg down to the floor, totally releasing all of the muscles of your right leg. Let the thigh, knee, and foot roll out to the right side. Repeat on the left side.

Bring your breath down into your legs and feet. Feel the hip sockets, thigh bones and muscles, knees, calves, shins, ankles, feet, and toes totally relax. Breathe and feel your entire body relax even deeper.

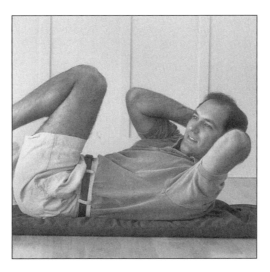

c h a p t e r   7

Firm the Abdominals and Trim the Waist

Do you ever feel . . .

. . . when you look for your toes, your waistline is in the way? Or has your waist disappeared completely in the folds of those "love handles"? There are abdominal muscles below those many layers of fat. Really there are. Our objective is to uncover those helpful muscles and activate them to define your waistline once again.

Here are a few abdominal yoga stretches to firm the abdominals and trim the waistline. Often lower back problems are caused by weak abdominal muscles pulling the lower back into a contracted position, resulting in lordosis (extreme lower back curve). This may also cause chronic tightness and disc problems. By strengthening the abdominals, you save your lower back from overworking. These postures will help you to create a balance of strength between the abdominal muscles in the front and the paraspinal muscles in the back of your body, which in turn will not only strengthen a flabby abdomen but decrease lower back problems.

! Caution: If you are pregnant, consult your doctor before doing any of the stretches in this chapter. Also, if you are menstruating, certain stretches are not recommended. Watch for additional caution notes in this section.

✔ Equipment Note: A yoga sticky mat and/or a blanket, and a chair.

Breathing with Retention (*Uddhiyana Bandha*)

Stand with your feet parallel and hip-width apart. Inhale and bring your arms out to your sides and over your head, filling your belly, ribs, and upper chest with air.

Exhale and slightly bend your legs, bringing the arms down by your sides, and place your hands on your thighs.

Release air from your belly, diaphragm, and lungs. Feel the navel move to the lower back as the belly moves in and up toward the ribs, pushing the last bit of breath out of your lungs. (See Figure 7.1, page 92.) Hold for a few seconds until you feel the need to take a breath in.

Relax the abdomen and allow your body to welcome your breath in once again.

Exhale and push the air out again, becoming aware of your abdominal area drawing inward, and hold the breath out until you need to take another breath in.

Repeat three to seven times.

This is actually the practice of a bandha known as Uddhiyana Bandha (stomach lock). After letting the breath out, you are contracting the front muscles of the abdomen and drawing them in, forming a hollow as you hold the breath out before taking the next breath in.

! **Caution:** If you are pregnant or are menstruating, **do not** practice this technique.

✔ **Elise's Note:** I like to think of it as pausing between breaths, finding total stillness rather than holding the breath out, which implies tension. As you do this regularly, you will find that you can hold the breath out longer. This not only strengthens a flabby abdomen but relieves constipation and indigestion.

✔ **Carol's Note:** Be sure not to overdo it. If you feel like you cannot hold the breath out comfortably any more, please take a breath in. No passing out allowed!

Stretching

Stomach Rolls

This exercise teaches you to identify and isolate your abdominal muscles so that you can begin to strengthen them.

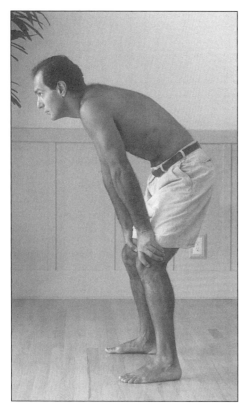

Figure 7.1
Feel the navel move to your lower back as you release air from your belly, diaphragm, and lungs

Stand with your feet parallel and hip-width apart. Keeping your arms at your sides, inhale and fill your belly, ribs, and upper chest with air.

Exhale and slightly bend your legs, placing your hands on your thighs above your knees, releasing air from your belly, diaphragm, and lungs. (See Figure 7.1.) Feel the navel move to the lower back as the belly moves in.

Pushing the last bit of breath out of your lungs, hold the breath out and pump the abdominal muscles in and out ten times. Be sure to not breathe as you pump your abdominals. Keeping the breath out creates more space for the pumping movements. As you pump in, pull the navel in and up toward the ribs. As you push out, let the abdominal muscles fully extend.

Inhale, relax the belly, and straighten the knees, coming up to a standing position.

Repeat this sequence two more times, building up to twenty-six times per sequence.

! Caution: If you are pregnant or are menstruating, **do not** practice this technique.

✔ Elise's Note: This not only tones the abdominal muscles, but also helps you to relax your internal organs and helps digestion and elimination.

Yoga Sit-ups

Lie down on your back, with your knees bent and your feet on the floor, hip-width apart. Be sure that your heels are directly under your knees. Place your hands with your fingertips at your hairline.

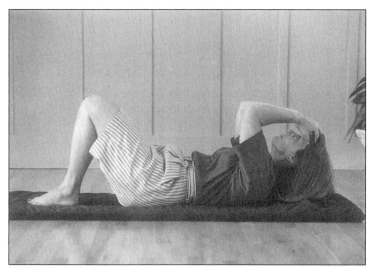

Figure 7.2
Draw your upper body toward your thighs, pressing your abdomen into your lower back

Inhale and exhale, drawing your upper body toward your thighs. (See Figure 7.2.) As you round your back, press your abdomen into your lower back, keeping your face parallel to the ceiling and not allowing your chin to move toward your chest. Feel your abdominal muscles contract.

Inhale and release your body back down to the floor. Exhale and lift again.

Repeat fifteen times, building up to fifty repetitions in one minute. Continue to breathe with each repetition.

At the end of your last inhalation, bring your body back down to the floor. To relax your abdomen, bring the bottoms of your feet together, letting your legs drop out to the floor.

Bring your arms up to shoulder height on the floor, with your elbows bent at a right angle and your palms facing the ceiling.

Take several deep breaths, relaxing the abdominal muscles and softening the abdominal area.

✔ **Elise's Note:** If this sit-up position irritates your lower back, place your feet on a wall with your legs at a right angle or rest your calves on the seat of a chair.

Leg Lifts (Urdhva Prasarita Padasana)

Lie on your back with your legs on the floor, stretching through your heels and your arms by your sides, palms pressing down.

Inhale and lift the right leg to the ceiling, perpendicular to the floor. Be sure that your lower back is in its neutral position.

On an exhalation, bring the leg down one third of the way to the floor. Breathe and hold this position.

Slowly lower your leg halfway to the floor. (See Figure 7.3, page 95.) Breathe and hold this position.

Lower your leg two-thirds of the way to the floor. Breathe and hold this position.

Finally, lower your leg a few inches from the floor. Breathe and hold this position.

Stretch through your heel and bring your leg down to the floor and relax. Repeat on the left side.

Variation One

As you increase your strength, stretch both arms overhead, with your palms facing the ceiling and your elbows straight.

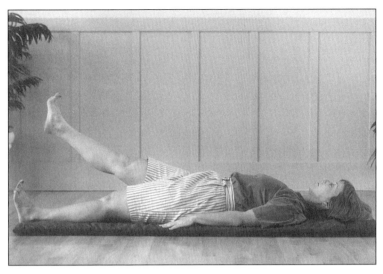

Figure 7.3
Pressing palms down, lower and hold your leg, remembering to breathe

Stretch from the hips through your fingertips. Repeat each leg lift sequence.

Variation Two

With your arms back at your sides, you can lift both legs at the same time, repeating the leg lift sequence. Be sure that you do not overcurve your lower back away from the floor and strain your lower back muscles.

To increase the difficulty, you may stretch your arms overhead as you lift and lower both legs, repeating the sequence.

If you feel any tightness in your lower back after doing this strengthener, draw your knees to your chest and bring your hands to your shins, stretching your lower back.

✔ **Elise's Note:** This leg lift strengthens the internal and external oblique muscles in your abdominal area. Be sure to not let your lower back overcurve from the floor. Think of pressing your lower back toward the floor as you bring the legs down to the floor. If you have lower back problems, bend the knee of the leg on the floor, placing your foot flat on the floor. This will help to keep the lower back from contracting.

✔ **Carol's Note:** These look easy but require abdominal strength. If you do a little at a time, you will get stronger. Hang in there.

Knee to Chest Abdominal

Lie down on your back, with your knees bent and your feet on the floor, hip-width apart. Be sure that your heels are directly under your knees. Bring your arms down by your sides, with your palms facing down.

Inhale and exhale, bringing the knees to the chest. (See Figure 7.4, page 97.) Inhale and stretch the legs up so that they are perpendicular to the floor, and extend through the heels.

Exhale and slowly bring the legs down to the floor just far enough to maintain the neutral position of your lower back. (See Figure 7.5, page 97.) If you feel your lower back rising, raise your legs slightly. Remember the position of your legs to begin the next movement.

Exhale, bringing your knees to your chest. Inhale and stretch your legs out again to the same position. Exhale and bring the knees back to your chest.

Breathe and repeat ten times, working up to thirty repetitions.

At the end of your last exhalation, bring your hands to your shins and continue to breathe, feeling a stretch in your lower back.

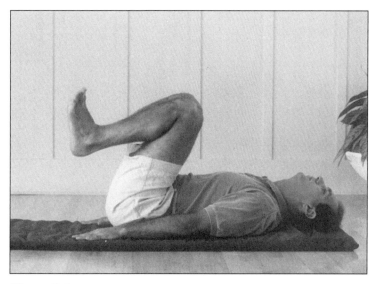

Figure 7.4
With your palms pressing down, bring the knees to the chest
as you exhale

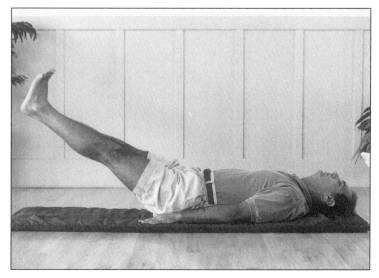

Figure 7.5
Inhale and slowly lower the legs just far enough to maintain
the neutral position of your lower back

To relax your abdomen, release your hands from your shins and bring your feet flat on the floor, with your knees bent.

Let the knees and thighs roll out to the side and bring the bottoms of your feet together. Place your arms up to shoulder height on the floor, with your elbows bent at a right angle and your palms facing the ceiling. Take several deep breaths, relaxing the abdominal muscles and softening the abdominal area.

Variation

As you increase your strength, stretch both arms overhead, with your palms facing the ceiling and your elbows straight. Stretch from the hips through your fingertips as you practice this sequence.

This abdominal strengthener is particularly good for anyone with lower back problems. It gives you a chance to recover by bringing your knees to your chest between each leg lift and also helps you to remember to breathe.

✔ **Elise's Note:** If you find the leg lifts with one leg too easy but with both legs too hard, practice this one for a while and you'll be able to build up to doing leg lifts with both legs and not hurting your back.

Cross Overs

Lie down on your back, with your knees bent and your feet on the floor, hip-width apart. Be sure that your heels are directly under your knees. Bring your arms down by your sides with your palms facing down.

Inhale and exhale, bringing the knees to the chest. Inhale, lifting your head slightly, and interlace your fingers behind your head.

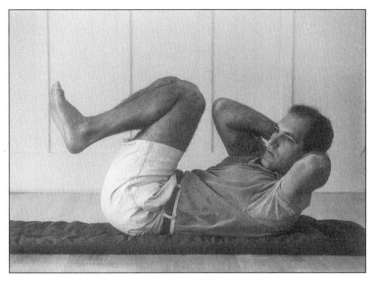

Figure 7.6
With your fingers interlaced behind your head, lift your head slightly and cross your right elbow over toward your left knee

Exhale and cross your right elbow over toward your left knee. (See Figure 7.6.)

Inhale and come back to your center, placing your head and upper body back on the floor.

Exhale and reverse, crossing your left elbow over to your right knee. This strengthens your transverse obliques that run diagonally across the abdominal area.

Repeat these cross overs ten times, building up to thirty.

At the end of your last exhalation, come back to your center and bring your hands to your shins. Continue to breathe, feeling a stretch in your lower back.

To relax your abdomen, release your hands from your shins and bring your feet flat to the floor, with your knees bent. Now let the knees and thighs roll out to the side and bring the bottoms of your feet together.

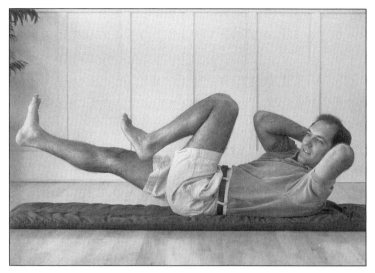

Figure 7.7
For a variation, as your right elbow crosses over to your left knee, stretch your right leg out, extending through the heel

Bring your arms up to shoulder height on the floor, with your elbows bent at a right angle and your palms facing the ceiling.

Take several deep breaths, relaxing the abdominal muscles and softening the abdominal area.

Variation One

As you increase your strength, keep your head and hands slightly off the floor as you come back to center between the cross overs.

Variation Two

As your right elbow crosses over to your left side, stretch your right leg out, extending through your heel. (See Figure 7.7.) Inhale and come back to center.

Exhale and reverse, crossing the left elbow to the right side and stretching your left leg out. This is the most challenging variation.

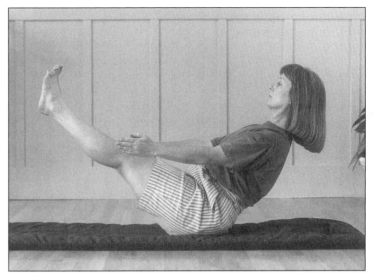

Figure 7.8
Lift the legs to sixty degrees from the floor, balancing on the front of your sitting bones; stretch out through your heels, keeping your lower back in its natural curve

Complete Boat Pose **(Paripurna Navasana)**

Sit in Staff or Rod Pose (see page 64 and Figure 8.9, page 119), with your legs together, stretched out in front of you. Bring your hands to your right buttock and move the flesh and skin out of the way so that you are sitting on your "sitting bones." Repeat on the left side.

Bend your knees with your feet flat on the floor. Place your index fingers at the creases under your knees and grasp your thighs. Inhale and lean your upper torso back thirty degrees (or one-third of the way) so that your arms straighten.

Remain on your sitting bones, exhale, and lift the legs to sixty degrees from the floor (two-thirds of the way), balancing on the front of your sitting bones. Stretch out through your heels, keeping your lower back in its natural curve. (See Figure 7.8.)

Breathe and slowly release your hands from your legs, stretching them out in front, with palms facing. Be sure to lengthen your spine toward your head, keeping your lower back in.

Stretch your legs toward your feet, keeping the knees and elbows straight. Lift the chest and look toward the feet.

Breathe and hold for twenty to thirty seconds. Holding this position for even a few breaths is beneficial.

Exhale and bring the legs back to the floor, relaxing in Staff or Rod Pose.

✔ **Elise's Note:** If you find it difficult to balance, bring your feet to a wall to gain more stability. This will also help you to lift your spine.

There is a tendency to hold the breath when doing this one, so be sure to keep breathing!

Half Boat Pose (Ardha Navasana)

Sit in Staff or Rod Pose (see page 64 and Figure 8.9, page 119), with your legs together, stretched out in front of you. Make sure you are sitting on your "sitting bones."

Bring the hands to the back of your head and interlace your fingers. Bend your knees and place your feet flat on the floor.

Exhale and lean your upper torso back, keeping your elbows forward. Raise the legs thirty degrees off the floor (one-third of the way) and balance, extending the spine and straightening the legs. (See Figure 7.9, page 103.)

Breathe and hold for fifteen to twenty seconds, looking toward your feet.

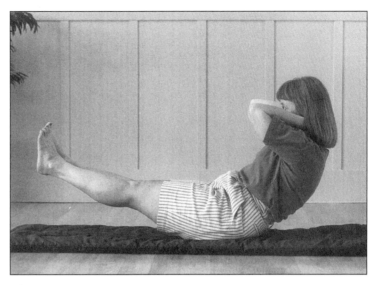

Figure 7.9
Raise the legs thirty degrees off the floor and balance,
extending the spine and straightening the legs

Slowly bring your legs back down to the
floor and release your hands, sitting in Staff
or Rod Pose.

✔ **Elise's Note:** Sometimes when you're first
getting the hang of this, you may roll down on
your back. Have no fear, just make sure you have
good padding beneath. Don't try to be perfect in
these poses, or you'll never improve. Just have fun
and laugh at yourself—it is very freeing.

Relaxation *(Savasana)*

Sitting in Staff or Rod Pose (see page 64 and
Figure 8.9, page 119), slowly round your
back as you lower your spine to the floor,
vertebra by vertebra. Use your abdominal
muscles to control your descent. Lie flat on
your back on the floor.

Align your head with the center of your body. If your chin is higher that your forehead, place a blanket under your head. Bring your arms down by your sides, forty-five degrees away from your thighs, to allow your shoulders to drop down to the floor.

You may record the rest on audio tape.

Inhale and make a fist with your hands. Squeeze your buttocks and lift your head, shoulders, arms and legs off the floor. Draw your shoulders up to your ears and contract your buttocks and abdomen, squeezing your entire body.

Exhale and drop your entire body to the floor. Be sure that your shoulders are dropped away from your ears and your back is relaxing into the floor.

Now feel all of your abdominal muscles totally relaxing. Feel all of the organs in your lower pelvis region relaxing. Imagine relaxing your stomach, intestines, liver, spleen, kidneys, and adrenal glands. As you feel your diaphragm softly rise and fall, focus on your breathing. As you inhale, feel your navel expand and as you exhale, feel all of your abdominal area soften and let go.

Invite peace and well-being into your mind and your entire body. When you are ready, take a deep breath, gently move your fingers and toes, and stretch out and open your eyes. Now bring your knees toward your chest, roll over to your side, and using your hands, push back up to a sitting position.

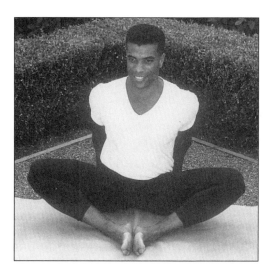

chapter 8

Stretch for Sports: Hamstrings, Quads, and Hips

Do you ever feel . . .

. . . your hamstrings are made of solid steel? The more you exercise, the tighter they become. You know you should stretch before and after exercising, but you are anxious to get on with it, so you skip the preparation stretches. And when you are finished, you've already spent all that time exercising, so why stretch any more? Also, as you get older, you may find that if you don't stretch, you run the risk of injuring yourself.

This chapter focuses on stretches that loosen up your body before and after exercising. Many people have very tight hamstrings and this can lead to lower back problems. The hamstrings are actually three muscles that form a large muscle group that runs from the back of the inner leg to the outer leg and attach from your buttocks to below your knee. When the hamstrings are tight, they pull on the lower back, bringing your lower back out of alignment, and often decreasing the curvature in your lower back. This also affects posture in your upper torso, which causes the chest to drop.

Stretching your hamstrings before exercising is a great injury-prevention policy. In many of these stretches, we are stretching the entire back of the leg, including the calf, down to the achilles tendon, which will prevent cramping in the back of the leg during and after exercising. When stretching the hamstrings, you will also feel the hips and buttocks areas being stretched since the hamstrings attach in the buttocks.

The quadricep muscle group in the front of the thigh is equally as important to stretch. Consisting of four muscles, this group is responsible for flexing the thigh to your chest as is the psoas muscle mentioned in Chapter 5. If this muscle becomes tight, it will affect your posture, thrusting you forward and creating too much of a lumbar curve (lordosis), resulting in chronic tightness in the lower back.

Once you learn these stretches, you can do them as a series, with one flowing into the next one. Ten minutes before and ten minutes after exercising is all you need to do. You will feel the difference.

✔ **Equipment Note:** A yoga sticky mat (if you're on a slippery surface or rug), a belt, a book or a yoga block, a blanket, a chair or a bench.

Breathing

Now that you are ready to go for your run (or start some other aerobic activity), it's time to energize your body with breathing.

Stand with your feet parallel, hip-width apart, with your hips over your heels and your arms down by your sides. Bring your arms behind you, interlacing your fingers, with the palms facing toward your back.

Inhale as you bring the arms up away from your buttocks. Stretch the shoulder blades together, opening the chest.

Exhale and release the arms down to your buttocks.

Repeat five times. Be sure to not lean forward or bend the elbows when you lift the arms behind you.

Now once again, inhale and lift the arms. Exhale and continue to breathe for four more breaths.

On the next exhalation, bend forward from your hips and allow the arms to raise high toward the sky or ceiling, and if possible, over the head. Stay in the position, taking five breaths in and out.

Inhale and raise your upper torso. Exhale and bring the arms down toward your buttocks and release the fingers.

Notice how much looser your shoulders are and how much more open your chest feels to take in deeper breaths. At the end, when you bend over, you get a bonus of stretching your hamstrings.

Stretching

Before Exercising

Right-Angled Wall Stretch
(*Ardha Uttanasana*)

Stand facing a wall or a railing, with your feet parallel, hip-width apart. Place your hands on the wall at hip level, with your head between your arms.

Walk your feet back so your hips are directly over your heels. Be sure your lower back is in its natural curve so that your buttocks bones are slightly higher than your lower back.

Inhale and spread your fingers, pressing the base of your thumb, index, and middle fingers into the wall as you stretch the pelvis back, lengthening your spine.

Exhale and push the shoulder blades down toward the floor. Your back should be parallel to the floor, forming a right angle with the lower body. (See Figure 8.1, page 109.) Breathe and hold for one minute.

Inhale, pressing your heels down to the floor as you lift your arms from the wall, bringing them over your head.

Exhale and bring them down by your sides.

✔ **Elise's Note:** If your hamstrings are tight and you cannot bring your lower back into its natural curve with your buttocks bones up, bend your knees to relieve your hamstrings and tilt your pelvis so that you feel your lower back move in. Slowly straighten your legs, lifting your thigh muscles, so that your lower back stays in its natural curve. If you still cannot bring your lower

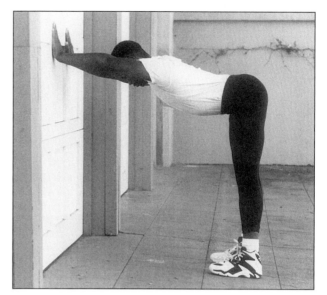

Figure 8.1
With your back parallel to the floor, push your
shoulder blades down

back in, walk your hands up to shoulder level and
do the pose with your hands at a higher position.

One-Legged Hamstring Stretch
(*Parvottanasana*)

Stand facing a wall or a railing, with your
feet parallel and hip-width apart. Place your
hands on the wall at hip level, with your
head between your arms.

Walk your feet back so that your hips are
directly over your heels. Be sure your lower
back is in its natural curve so that your buttocks bones are slightly higher than your
lower back.

Inhale and bring your right foot forward
eighteen inches. Exhale and bring your left
foot back eighteen inches, making sure your
right heel is in line with your left heel. (See
Figure 8.2, page 110.)

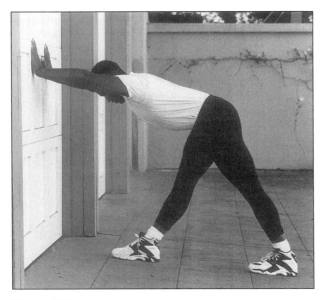

Figure 8.2
Make sure your hips are level as you stretch them
back while pressing with your palms

Bring your right hand to your buttocks to
make sure they are level. If the right buttock
is higher, bring the right foot forward. If the
left buttock is higher, slide the left foot back.

Bring your hand back to the wall and press
with your inner palms, stretching your hips
back. Breathe and hold for one minute.

Exhale and bring your feet back together in
the right-angle stretch position. Repeat on
the opposite side.

To increase the stretch in the hamstrings,
raise the ball of the front foot, flexing the toes
toward the shin and lifting the thigh muscle.
Feel the hip of the front leg moving back.
Keep the hip moving back as you slowly
bring the foot back down to the floor.

✔ **Elise's Note:** This is a great upper hamstring,
hips, and buttocks stretch to do before exercising.
Even though it is called One-Legged Hamstring
Stretch, you can also feel the stretch in the hamstrings and calf muscle of the back leg.

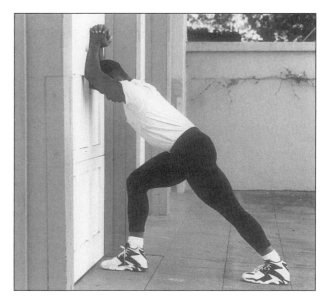

Figure 8.3
Feel the stretch from your forearms, through your chest, down your left leg, to your calf and heel

Calf and Quad Stretch

Stand facing a wall and bring your right foot to the wall. Place your left foot behind four and one-half feet, with the right heel in line with your left heel.

Bend your right leg to form a right angle, with your knee over your heel. If the calf or quadricep is tight, you may not be able to form a right angle at first; just keep stretching and it will happen.

Interlace your fingers and stretch your arms over your head, placing your forearms on the wall. (See Figure 8.3.) Feel the stretch from your forearms, through your chest, down your left leg, to your calf and heel.

Breathe and hold for thirty seconds.

Now, to stretch the quadriceps in your back leg, release your fingers and bring your fingertips to the wall at shoulder level.

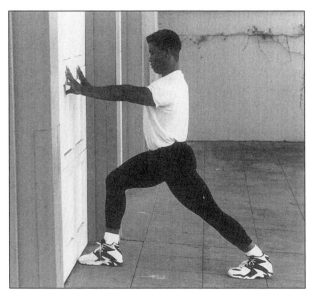

Figure 8.4
As you stretch back through the heel, be sure your right leg continues to form a right angle

Drop your shoulders, tuck the pelvis, and press your fingertips into the wall, straightening your arms, making sure that your upper body is directly over your hips.

Stretch back through your left heel to feel the stretch in your quadriceps in the left front thigh. (See Figure 8.4.) Be sure that your right leg continues to bend, forming a right angle.

Breathe and hold thirty seconds.

Inhale, straighten your right leg and bring your feet back together.

Repeat on the opposite side.

✔ **Elise's Note:** When doing the quadricep stretch, you may want to use a mirror in the beginning to make sure your upper body is directly over the hips. If you're not feeling the stretch, you are probably leaning too far forward or not tucking the buttocks enough.

This quadricep stretch also stretches the psoas muscle, which relieves your lower back, as did the Kneeling Lunge. (See Figure 5.7, page 59.)

Shooting Bow Pose *(Natarajasana)*

Standing eight inches away from the wall, feet parallel and hip-width apart, inhale and stretch your arms over your head and place on the wall.

Exhale and bend your left knee, grasping the ankle, flexing the toes toward your shin, and stretching through your heel.

Stretch down through the left thigh toward the floor, bringing your left knee back and in line with your right leg. Remember to tuck your buttocks so that your tailbone moves toward the front of your body.

Like a shooting bow, pull your heel back away from your buttocks, flexing your foot, keeping your left knee hip-width apart. Breathe and stretch your right arm up the wall, lifting the left thigh so that your leg lifts up toward the ceiling. (See Figure 8.5.)

Exhale and release your hand from your foot, bringing it back to the floor.

Repeat on the opposite side.

This stretches the quadriceps and psoas muscle and prepares you to begin back bends.

Standing Hamstring Stretch *(Utthita Hasta Padangusthasana)*

Stand in Palm Tree Pose (see Figure 2.8, page 18) facing a short fence, railing, or counter top.

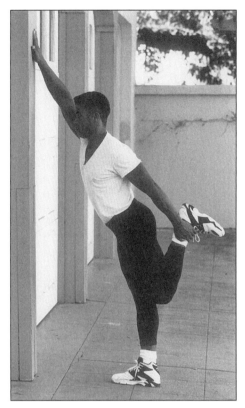

Figure 8.5
Stretch your arm up the wall as you lift your thigh

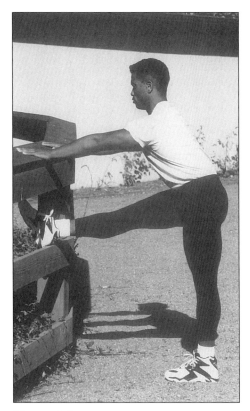

Figure 8.6
Keep your legs straight as you bend from the hips

Inhale, and on exhalation, raise the right leg to place your right foot on the fence, keeping the left leg firm. Keep your left foot facing forward and your hips parallel.

Keeping the left leg straight, stretch through your right heel, straightening the leg.

Inhale and stretch your arms over your head. Exhale and stretch your arms down, placing your hands on the fence (see Figure 8.6.), or grab the ball of your right foot. If you cannot reach your foot, use a belt to place around the ball of your foot, holding the ends of the belt in your hands. Be sure to lift through your spine and bend from your hips, rather than rounding your back and bending your forehead to your leg.

Breathe and hold for thirty seconds and build up to one minute.

Inhale and release the hold, bringing the arms over your head. Exhale and bring your right foot to the floor, bringing your arms to your sides.

Repeat on the opposite side.

✔ **Elise's Note:** If you cannot reach a fence or counter, use a chair or a bench in the beginning.

✔ **Carol's Note:** This is a "for real" hamstring stretch.

Standing Inner Thigh Stretch
(Utthita Hasta Padangusthasana)

Stand in Palm Tree Pose (see Figure 2.8, page 18), with your right side toward the fence and leg-width away from the fence.

Place your right heel on the fence, in line with your left foot. Place both hands on your hips.

Inhale, and on exhalation, slide the right hand down the right leg, reaching with your index and middle fingers toward your big toe. If you cannot reach your toe, use a belt or place your right hand on your shin.

Keeping your hips parallel and your left leg straight, stretch out through your right heel, straightening your leg and aligning your body.

Inhale and turn the palm of your left hand to the ceiling or sky. Exhale and stretch the left arm up and over your head, stretching your left hand toward the fence.

Breathe and hold for thirty seconds, building up to one minute.

Inhale and release the hold, bringing the arms over your head. Exhale and bring your right foot to the floor, bringing your arms to your sides.

Repeat on the opposite side.

✔ **Elise's Note:** If you cannot reach a fence or counter, use a chair or a bench in the beginning. This pose stretches the inner thighs called the adductor muscles.

Wide-Angled Standing Pose (*Prasarita Padottanasana*)

Stand in Palm Tree Pose (see Figure 2.8, page 18), with your feet four and one-half to five feet apart. Stretch the thighs up and roll your weight to the outer heels so your weight is centered on both feet.

Bring your hands to the crease where your legs meet your torso, placing your forefingers in front and your thumbs at your sides. Inhale and lift up through your spine.

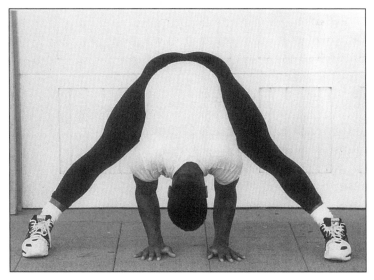

Figure 8.7
If you can bring your palms flat, walk your hands back to line
up your fingers with your toes

Exhale and bend over at your hips, dropping your upper body to the floor. Keep your thighs lifted and your knees straight.

Slowly release your hands, placing your fingertips or palms on the floor directly under your shoulders, shoulder-width apart. (See Figure 8.7.)

If you can bring your palms flat, walk your hands back to line up your fingers with your toes.

Bend the elbows back, keeping the elbows shoulder-width apart. Release your neck and head. Be sure to stretch your inner legs and thighs out away from each other.

Breathe and hold for thirty seconds.

Bring your hands back to the tops of your legs. Inhale and extend your spine as you come up halfway, with your upper body parallel to the floor.

To lift the upper body completely to a vertical position, press down through your heels, lifting through your thighs. Feel the support through your legs as you tuck the buttocks under when you come up.

This pose stretches the inner hamstrings and inner thighs (adductor muscles) and also relieves the pelvis, sacrum, and lower back.

After Exercising

Standing Forward Bend (Uttanasana)

Stand in Palm Tree Pose (see Figure 2.8, page 18), with your feet hip-width apart. Bring your hands to the crease where your legs meet your torso, placing your forefingers in front and your thumbs at your sides. Inhale, lifting up through your spine.

Exhale and bend over at your hips, dropping your upper body to the floor. Keep your thighs lifted and your knees straight.

Slowly release your hands and bring your fingertips to the floor in front of your feet. Bring some weight forward into the balls of your feet and your fingers. Keep your hips and ankles in line. (See Figure 8.8.)

Release your abdomen, neck, and head. Breathe and hold for thirty seconds.

Bring your hands back to the tops of your legs. Inhale and extend your spine as you come up halfway, with your upper body parallel to the floor. Exhale and bring the lower back into its natural curve.

Inhale and lift the upper body to a vertical position, pressing down through your heels, lifting through your thighs, feeling the support through your legs.

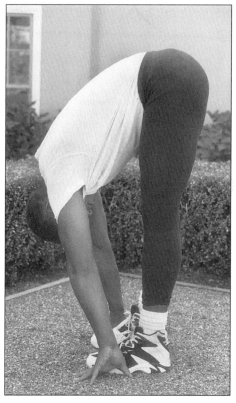

Figure 8.8
Bring some weight forward into the balls of your feet and fingers

For a deeper stretch of the hamstrings, if your hands can reach the floor, place your fingers on the outsides of your feet, in line with your toes.

✔ **Elise's Note:** An important part of this posture is coming back up. This is the best training to learn to use your legs to lift your upper back. If you are bending from your waist and feel your lower back rounding, repeat Right-Angled Wall Stretch. (See Figure 8.1, page 109.) If you cannot quite reach the floor, press your fingers into a book or yoga block to deepen your stretch and align your body.

Wide-Angled Sitting Pose
(Upavistha Konasana)

Sit on the floor with your legs together, stretched out in front of you. Bring your hands to your right buttock and move the flesh and skin out of the way so that you are sitting on your "sitting bones." Repeat on the left side.

If your lower back is rounded, sit on the edge of a folded blanket to help you correctly position your lower back.

Take a breath in and lift the arms to your sides and overhead. Exhale and continue to breathe as you keep the lift of the back, maintaining all four natural curves of the spine. Lift from the lower back, engaging all the muscles of the back.

Bring the arms down by your sides, lift up through your spine, and stretch out through your heels, pressing your thighs to the floor. (See Figure 8.9, page 119.) This is called Staff or Rod Pose and is a wonderful back strengthener in itself.

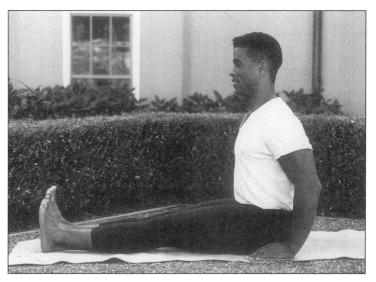

Figure 8.9
Stretching out through your heels, press your thighs to
the floor

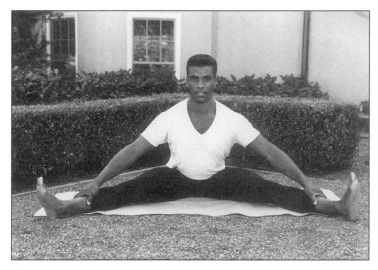

Figure 8.10
If you can bend forward, put your hands on your shins . . .
if not, keep your hands behind you

Spread your legs out to the sides, keeping the knees and toes facing up to the ceiling. Bring your hands behind you, pressing down with your hands and thighs, continuing to lift your spine.

Breathe and lean forward with your upper body for thirty seconds. If you can bend forward from your hips, place your hands on your shins or grab your big toes. (See Figure 8.10, page 119.)

Inhale, lift your arms overhead, bringing your upper body to an upright position. Exhale and bring your legs together.

This stretches your inner hamstrings and inner thighs (adductor muscles) as well as strengthens the back when you lift the arms overhead.

Bound Angle Pose (Baddha Konasana)

Sit on the floor with your legs together, stretched out in front of you. Bring your hands to your right buttock and move the flesh and skin out of the way so that you are sitting on your "sitting bones." Repeat on the left side.

If your lower back is rounded, sit on the edge of a folded blanket to help you correctly position your lower back.

Bring the arms down by your sides, lift up through your spine and stretch out through your heels, pressing your thighs to the floor. To get more lift and to strengthen the back, you may lift the arms overhead and breathe. This is called Staff or Rod Pose.

Bend your knees while bringing the bottoms of your feet together, sliding your heels in toward your body. Grab your ankles, pulling your heels in closer to your body. If your lower back is rounded, place your hands in

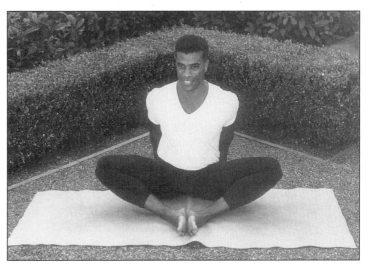

Figure 8.11
Grab your ankles to pull your heels in closer, or if your lower back rounds, put your hands behind you

back of you on the floor, pressing down with your hands to lift your spine. (See Figure 8.11.)

Press through your heels, lengthening your thighs from your hips to your knees, dropping your knees toward the floor.

If your lower back is in its natural curve and not rounded, you may interlace your fingers around your toes and lift the spine, bending forward from your hips.

Press your elbows to your thighs to bring your legs farther down to the floor.

Breathe and hold for one minute.

Release your hands and straighten your legs.

✔ **Elise's Note:** If you're seated high on one or more blankets and cannot reach the floor behind you to get the lift of the spine without rounding, place two blocks or books behind you, placing your hands on them to get a better lift.

✔ **Carol's Note:** If you hadn't noticed, this really stretches your inner thighs and your groin. Don't worry if your knees are pointing toward your nose when you start. Just keep practicing.

Sitting Hip Opener

Sit on the floor with your legs together, stretched out in front of you. Bring the arms down by your sides, lift up through your spine and stretch out through your heels, pressing your thighs to the floor. If your lower back is rounded, sit on the edge of a folded blanket to help you correctly position your lower back.

Bend both knees slightly, bringing your feet flat on the floor. Place your hand on your left shin, drawing your leg toward you, passing the left foot under your right thigh.

Use your right hand to turn your foot so that the top is placed on the floor and the bottom of your foot points toward the ceiling. Your left heel should be next to your right buttock.

Pick up the right leg and place it on top of the left leg so that the knees are in line. Place the top of your right foot on the floor so that the bottom of your foot points toward the ceiling. Your right heel is next to your left buttock. (See Figure 8.12, page 123.)

If your knees are off the floor and your back is rounded, use additional pillows or blankets to raise your buttocks. This will help you to drop your knees to the floor to deepen your hip stretch.

Place your fingertips on the floor behind your hips. Inhale and lift your spine and rib cage from your pelvis.

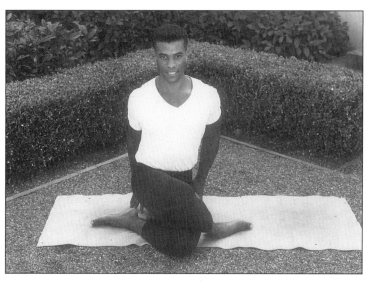

Figure 8.12
Place your hands behind you as you inhale and lift the spine and rib cage from your pelvis

Exhale and drop your buttocks bones. Your spine should be in an upright alignment, with your lower back in a natural curve.

Breathe and hold for one minute. Place blocks behind you if you are high on a blanket and lift with your hands on the blocks.

To deepen the stretch, slowly come forward, placing your ribs on your thighs. Inhale and reach your arms out in front of you, with your palms on the floor, stretching your entire back.

Breathe and hold for thirty seconds.

Another variation is to use your hands to move your ankles out in line with your knees. Hold your ankles and breathe for thirty seconds. Uncross your legs and repeat on the other side.

This hip opener stretches all the muscles in the buttocks, particularly the piriformis muscle, which helps to relieve sciatica.

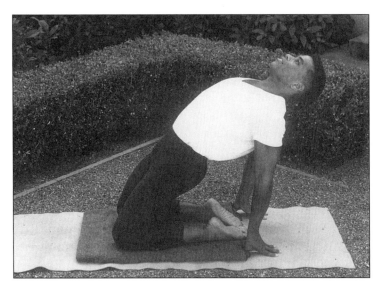

Figure 8.13
Lift the chest toward the ceiling as you squeeze the buttocks
and stretch your thighs

Kneeling Thigh Stretch *(Ustrasana)*

This is a flowing stretch where the body and breath
move together.

> Kneel down and sit back on your heels, with
> the tops of your feet on the floor and big toes
> touching. Be sure that the knees are hip-
> width apart.

> Place your fingers on the floor behind your
> hips. Exhale and squeeze the buttocks, lifting
> the pelvis from your heels and stretching
> your thighs forward.

> Inhale and lift the chest toward the ceiling.
> (See Figure 8.13.) Exhale and bring the but-
> tocks back down to the heels. Inhale and lift
> the spine.

> Exhale and stretch forward into Child's Pose
> (see page 53), bringing the chest to the thighs.
> Allow your forehead to rest on the floor, let-
> ting your arms relax by your sides. (See Figure
> 8.14, page 125.)

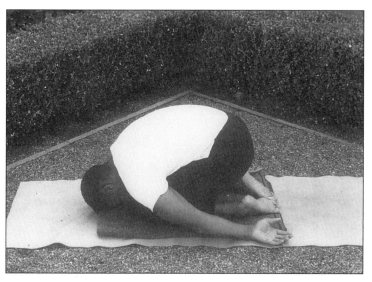

Figure 8.14
Lean forward into Child's Pose, bringing the chest to the thighs and forehead to the floor

Inhale and come back up, sitting on your heels. Exhale and lift the buttocks again, expanding the chest.

Inhale, stretch the thighs forward, opening the front body farther. Exhale and bring the buttocks to the heels and come forward into Child's Pose again.

You can repeat this five times or more.

On the last one, hold the thigh stretch for five breaths, getting a deeper stretch.

If you are more flexible with this thigh stretch, grab hold of your ankles.

This is a back bend that beginners can do. It opens the thoracic (mid-back) spine and stretches the quadriceps. It also helps decrease rounded shoulders and kyphosis (rounded mid-back).

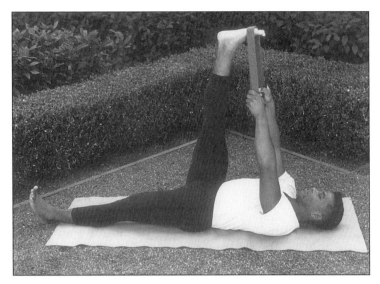

Figure 8.15
Slowly straighten your right leg while holding the belt, making sure to stretch through your right heel

Hamstring Stretch on the Floor with a Belt (*Supta Padangusthasana*)

Lie on your back with your legs straight and feet together, stretching through your heels. Place a blanket under your head if your chin is higher than your forehead.

Part one: Keeping your left leg firmly on the floor, lift your right leg toward the ceiling. Place your left hand on your left thigh.

Bend the right knee and place your belt around the ball of your foot. Inhale, pressing the left thigh down to the floor.

As you exhale, slowly straighten your right leg, holding your belt with one or both hands. (See Figure 8.15.)

Be sure that you are stretching through your right heel to stretch the back of your leg. Keep your shoulders down and the head straight.

Breathe and hold for thirty seconds.

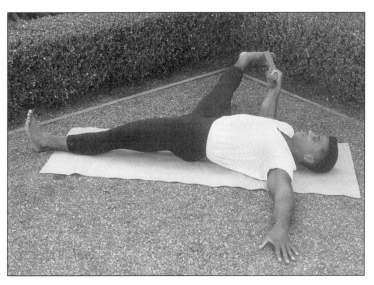

Figure 8.16
Keep the left side of the body firmly on the floor as you stretch out to the right

Inhale, then exhale, sliding your left hand down toward your knee and lift the head, shoulders, and upper body toward the right thigh. Hold and breathe for five breaths.

On an exhalation, release your spine and head back down to the floor.

Part one is the ultimate hamstring stretch for lower back problems.

Part two: Inhale and stretch up through your right leg. Hold the belt now in your right hand. Exhale, moving the right leg out toward the right side and down to the floor. (See Figure 8.16.)

Keep the left side of the body firmly on the floor as you continue to stretch out through the right side. Be sure to keep your right knee straight. If the left side lifts up off of the floor, raise the right leg slightly and press the left palm into your front left hip to secure the left side to the floor.

Breathe and hold for thirty seconds.

Inhale and lift your right leg back up toward the sky and remove the belt from your foot. Exhale and bring your leg down to the floor and relax.

Repeat this sequence on the opposite side.

Part two is great for stretching the inner thighs (adductor muscles).

Relaxation *(Savasana)*

You may record this on audio tape.

Lie flat on your back on the floor. Align your head with the center of your body. If your chin is higher than your forehead, place a blanket under your head.

Bring your arms down by your sides, forty-five degrees away from your thighs to allow your shoulders to drop down to the floor. Be sure your shoulders drop away from your ears.

Inhale, and on exhalation make an "ahhhh" sound, letting the whole body sink into the floor. Begin to feel your whole body from your head through your toes letting go.

Feel the muscles in your arms and legs relaxing even deeper and deeper. Visualize your muscles relaxing away from your bones. Feel your buttock muscles relaxing away from the pelvis. Feel the quadriceps releasing from the thigh bones. Feel the inner thigh muscles releasing from the thigh bones. Feel the hamstrings releasing from the thigh bones. Feel the calf muscles relaxing away from the shin bones. Feel all of the muscles in your feet relaxing away from all of the small bones. Continue to breathe as you let all of your leg muscles relax even deeper.

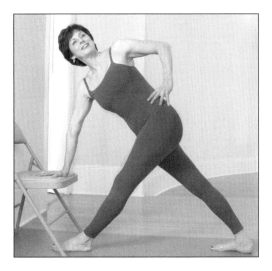

chapter 9

Strengthen and Stretch with Classic Yoga Poses

Do you ever feel . . .

You want to strengthen and stretch your whole body, and build your confidence in practicing more classic yoga poses at home?

Without going to a regular yoga class, you can follow the step-by-step process presented in this chapter to learn how to do poses that are often presented in a class of more seasoned yoga students.

To continue learning more classic yoga poses, using props can help you build confidence. We show you a step-by-step way to work up to more classic yoga poses with the assistance from props.

These classic yoga poses add to your repertoire of the basic poses already presented in the other chapters.

In this chapter, we will show you how to focus on and lengthen your spine while strengthening your back muscles. You can use props to begin the learning process. As you learn the correct alignment, your practice can become more intense and you can hold each pose for the maximum benefit. All of these classic poses are taught with a therapeutic use of props. You can then progress at your own pace. Breaking down the poses and then building your strength results in a deeper practice. We recommend that you hold each pose for more than twenty seconds up to one minute to create the maximum stretch for greater strength and flexibility.

✔ **Equipment Note:** A chair, a block, a towel, a strap and a wall space. Use a sticky mat if you're on a slippery surface, such as a rug, so you don't slide in some of the stretches that require traction.

"In the work of Pranayama, the back is the blackboard, the air comes to write, and the mind holds the chalk."
—*B.K.S. Iyengar*

Breathing Pranayama

Now that you are ready to begin a more advanced practice, you can use one technique in the selection of the classic yoga breathing techniques called Pranayama introduced to you in Chapters 1 and 2.

Sit in a cross-legged position on the floor or sit in a dining room or folding chair. If you choose to sit cross legged, be sure to sit on folded blankets so that you can create a lift in your spine, can keep your lower back in its natural curve, and can prevent back and knee injury.

To keep your chest lifted, shoulders back and your body aligned, place your hands on a blanket or small pillow resting in your lap. Be sure to keep your upper arms in line with the sides of your body. Gently drop your chin towards your chest to create a "throat lock" (bandha) without dropping your chest.

Inhale and begin to observe your breath flowing in to your front ribs and chest. Exhale and gently release your breath from your lungs, keeping your rib cage and chest lifted. As you focus on your next inhalation, imagine your breath rising to your collarbone and descending to your diaphram simultaneously. Exhale and release your breath first from your lungs, followed by your ribs.

Maintain your focus on your vertical breaths. Next, allow your breath to expand laterally into your side ribs. Inhale and feel the expansion. Exhale and feel your release from your lungs and side ribs. If this is difficult to feel, you may place your hands on your side ribs and use pressure to move your breath in this region.

Now inhale and bring the conciousness of your breath to your back ribs and lungs. With an exhalation, softly release your breath from your lungs and back ribs without dropping your back.

To feel this complete breath in all areas, begin to inhale in to your back ribs, wrap your breath around to your side ribs and finish the inhalation with your breath rising and descending simultaneously. Exhale and release your breath from the back, side and front ribs as if deflating a balloon from all directions. Slowly increase the length of your breaths without straining or becoming tense. Gently bring your chin up and allow your breath to come back to normal.

Option with Belt

To keep your back from rounding and to maintain good posture, you may use a yoga strap. Loop the strap around your upper arms just above your elbows so that the strap presses across your back to lift your chest. Be sure that your upper arms and elbows line up with the sides of your body.

✔ **Elise's Note:** The goal is to have an even, smooth and equal inhalation and exhalation. This balances bringing your body energy and while maintaining calm.

Stretching with Classic Yoga Poses

Gate Pose (Parighasana)

This classic pose stretches the side body and releases tightness in the lower back.

Preparation Pose with a Chair

Find a dining room chair or a folding chair and kneel with your right side toward the seat of the chair approximately one leg's distance away. Place your right foot between the front two legs of the chair, with your right heel in line with your left knee. Make sure your left hip is directly in line with your left knee. Place your left hand on your left waist and your right hand at the top of your right thigh. Use your right thumb and index finger to press your thigh down, creating a fold in your leg to even up your hips.

Externally rotate your right thigh so that it moves towards the ceiling. Lift your right thigh and lengthen your right foot towards

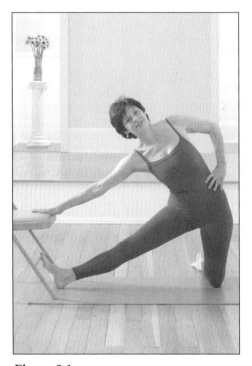

Figure 9.1
Make sure your left hip is in line with your left knee

the floor so that the ball of your foot and toes touch the floor. If your foot does not rest comfortably on the floor, you may place a towel or block under the ball of your foot.

Inhale and begin pressing with your right thumb and index finger into your thigh to create more of a fold as your hips move towards the left. As your upper body moves your right leg, reach your right hand out towards the chair and place your hand on the seat of the chair. Stretch out through your right side, lengthening the right side of your ribs and upper body. (See Figure 9.1, page 132.) Twist your right ribs towards the left to open your chest and align your shoulders. Breathe and hold the pose for thirty seconds up to one minute.

Inhale, press down through the left leg, release your right hand from the chair and bring your upper body back to center. Repeat on the opposite side.

Classic Pose

As you advance, you may eliminate the chair and use a block instead. Begin the pose with the same instructions as above, positioning a block next to the right side of your right ankle. As you reach out to lengthen your spine, place your right hand on the block for a greater stretch and twist your right ribs towards the left to open your chest. Bring your left arm out to your side with your palm facing up. Inhale and stretch your arm overhead. With an exhalation, stretch your arm towards the right, creating a diagonal line from your left knee through to your fingertips. (See Figure 9.2.) Feel the stretch of your left waist and ribs.

Hold the pose, increasing your time to one minute. Inhale and release coming back to

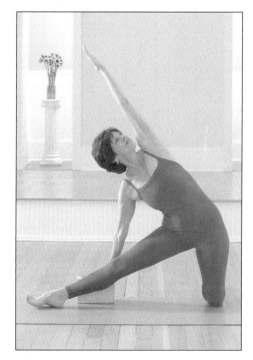

Figure 9.2
Place your right hand on the block for a greater stretch

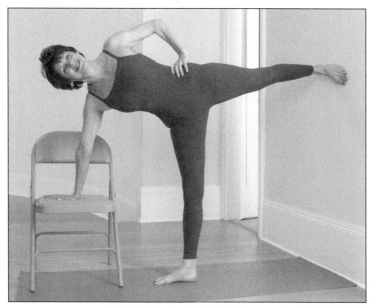

Figure 9.3
Draw the right buttocks forward and the left hip towards the
ceiling, revolving the lower abdomen and ribs up

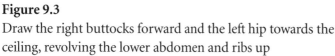

center. Repeat on the left side, repositioning the block next to the left side of your left ankle.

✔ **Elise's Note:** This pose is good for tightness of the lower back, to release back tension, and to increase your lung capacity for deeper breathing.

Half Moon (Ardha Chandrasana)

We introduced you to Triangle Pose, Trikonasana, in Chapter 6: Change Fat to Firm. You might have practiced this pose when you were working on strengthening and firming your legs and thighs. Now you will use Triangle Pose to approach a more advanced pose that will increase your balance as you extend your spine, arms and legs.

Preparation Pose with a Chair

Select a wall space and find a dining room or folding chair. Place the chair on your right side approximately four feet away from the wall. Place your left outer heel at the wall with your left foot slightly in toward the center of your body. Bring your right foot to a three and half feet distance from the wall with your right heel in line with the instep of your left foot.

Externally rotate your thighs away from each other so that the right knee is facing the ceiling and the left knee faces forward. Exhale and bend sideways towards the right leg, placing the right palm on the lower leg, forming a triangle.

Inhale, bend your right knee, and reach forward and place your right hand on the seat of the chair. Now exhale, bring the left foot slightly in towards the right foot and lift your left leg, placing your left foot flat on the wall at hip level. Make sure that your toes are turned slightly towards the floor. Draw the right buttocks forward and the left hip towards the ceiling, revolving the lower abdomen and ribs up. (See Figure 9.3, page 134.) Be sure to align your left hip with your left outer ankle. This will create an alignment and openness of the whole body. Stretch the left arm up towards the ceiling. Breathe and hold the pose for thirty seconds working up to one minute.

On an exhalation, bend your right knee, bringing your left foot back to the floor, placing the outer heel at the wall, going back into Triangle pose. Take several breaths, then press down through your legs and feet and come up to a standing position.

You will also feel this pose stretch the upper arm and armpit and open the chest. It also increases flexibility in the shoulder joint and brings the tips of the shoulder blades in toward the chest, realigning the upper body.

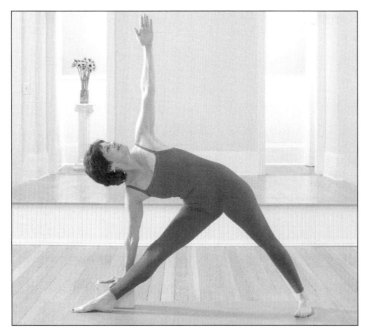

Figure 9.4
Bend your trunk sideways to the right, reaching your right
hand to the block at the outer ankle

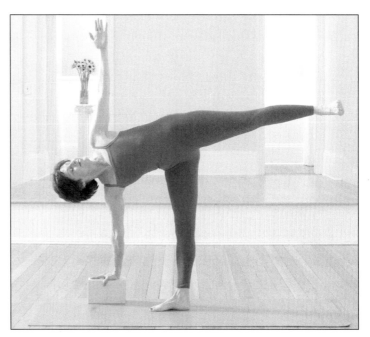

Figure 9.5
Feel the extension in opposite directions as you lengthen
your spine through the crown of your head

Classic Pose

As you advance, you may eliminate the chair and use a block instead, positioning yourself in the middle of the room. This one is going to require more strength and balance.

Place the block on your right side, stand in Palm Tree Pose (See Figure 2.8, page 18.) Place your feet four feet apart. Stretch your arms to the sides and turn your left foot slightly in and your right leg ninety degrees out. With an exhalation, bend your trunk sideways to the right, reaching your right hand to the block at the outer ankle and go into Triangle Pose. (See Figure 9.4, page 136.)

Exhale and bend your right knee, bringing your left foot slightly in towards your right foot. Holding the block, push the block forward and lift your left leg up towards the ceiling. Align your right hand and right shoulder with your left shoulder and hand, which you are extending towards the ceiling. Be firm on your right foot as you pull up through your right thigh. Extend your left leg through to your heel. Feel the extension in opposite directions as you lengthen your spine through the crown of your head. (See Figure 9.5, page 136.)

Remember to revolve your lower abdomen, lifting your left hip and keeping your left hip aligned with the left ankle. As you advance, you may complete the pose by turning your head towards the ceiling, looking at your left hand. Breathe and hold the pose for twenty to thirty seconds working up to one minute.

Exhale and bend your right knee and lower your left leg. Straighten your right leg and go back into Triangle pose. Make sure your feet are in the correct alignment and correct distance apart. Inhale and come up out of Triangle pose. Repeat on the opposite side.

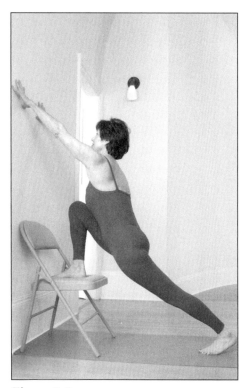

Figure 9.6
Extend through your back leg, pressing your outer heel to the floor

✔ **Elise's Note:** If your balance is an issue, you may place your left hand on your left hip to come into the pose or have your back at a wall for support.

✔ **Carol's Note:** This pose is a saying YES to life. It is impossible to be depressed in this pose.

Warrior One (Virabhadrasana One)

This is a widely recognized classic yoga pose. As is indicated in the name, this standing pose declares power and strength involving the whole body. It stretches the front of the body and can help you prepare for classic back bends.

Preparation Pose with a Chair

Find a dining room or folding chair. Place the chair at a wall and facing the chair, stand in Palm Tree Pose approximately three feet away from the seat of the chair. Bend your right knee and place your right foot on the seat of the chair. Bring your right knee directly over your right ankle and move your left foot slightly out to an eighty degree angle. Stretch your arms overhead and place your hands on the wall. Extend through your back leg, pressing your outer heel to the floor. As you extend your side ribs towards your arms, feel the stretch in your back muscles and your spine while opening your chest. (See Figure 9.6.) Breathe and feel the stretch in opposite directions. This also stretches the front of your back thigh and your psoas muscle. Hold the pose for thirty seconds building up to one minute.

Inhale, lift your arms overhead and feel the stretch in this position. Then press your right foot down and lift it off the chair

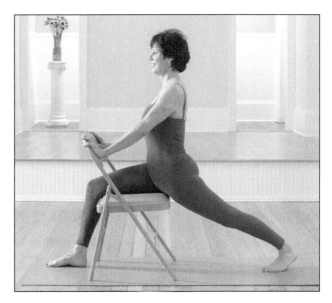

Figure 9.7
Draw your navel towards the lower back to align your hips, shoulders, ears and the crown of your head

coming back to Palm Tree Pose. Repeat on the opposite side.

Optional Pose with a Folding Chair

Place a folding chair the middle of the room. Stand facing the seat of the chair in Palm Tree Pose. Bring your right leg through the chair opening and place your right foot flat on the floor behind the back legs of the chair. Your right thigh will be resting on the seat of the chair and your left leg is extending back through the heel.

Bring the left hip forward so that it is parallel to the right hip. Press your hands into the back of the chair as you draw your navel towards the lower back to align your hips, shoulders, ears and the crown of your head. Your left heel may come off the floor. Remember to stretch through the back of your heel. (See Figure 9.7.)

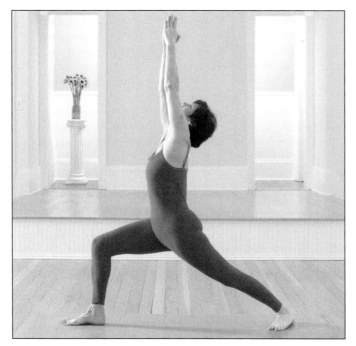

Figure 9.8
Be sure that your right knee is directly over your right ankle

Draw your tailbone down as you lift your inner left thigh and knee towards the ceiling. You should feel the stretch in your front left thigh and groin as you attempt to lift your right thigh off the seat of the chair. Engage your muscles to strengthen as you stretch.

Breathe and stretch for thirty seconds working up to one minute. Release your left leg and bring it to the side of the chair and stand up, bringing your right leg out of the back of the chair. Repeat on the opposite side.

Classic Pose

Stand in Palm Tree Pose. Bring the legs four to four and one half feet apart with the arms stretching to the sides, palms facing up. Inhale and stretch your arms over your head until they are parallel. Lift the sides of your ribs and chest. Turn your left foot forty-five to sixty degrees inward and your right foot ninety degrees outward.

With an exhalation, turn your torso to face your right leg. Inhale and lift your spine and upper torso towards the ceiling while you firmly press your back heel into the floor. With an exhalation, bend your right knee to create a right angle with your thigh. Be sure that your right knee is directly over your right ankle. Draw your navel towards your lower back and draw your tailbone down to keep your pelvis parallel to the floor. (See Figure 9.8, page 140.) Hold the pose for twenty to thirty seconds, breathing evenly.

Inhale and press down with your right foot as you straighten your right leg. Bring your feet parallel and lower your arms to return to Palm Tree Pose.

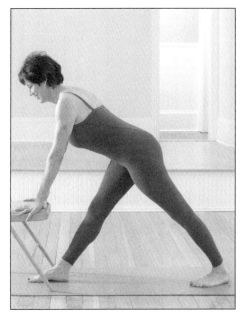

Figure 9.9
Draw back through your hips as you extend forward through your spine

One-Legged Hamstring Stretch (Parsvottanasana)

We introduced you to One-Legged Hamstring Stretch in Chapter 8: Stretch for Sports. You might have practiced this pose when you were working on stretching your hamstrings, quads and hips. Now you will use this pose to improve your balance and open your chest to energize your whole upper and lower body.

Preparation Pose with a Chair

Find a dining room or folding chair. Place the chair directly in front of you. Position your right foot between the front legs of the chair and bring your left foot three and one half feet behind your the right foot. Line up your right heel and left heel with your left foot turned in seventy-five degrees. Place your hands on your hips and bring your left hip in line with your right hip.

Inhale and lift your chest, bringing your side ribs up out of your pelvis. Spread your collarbone horizontally and draw your elbows back. Exhale and fold forward from your hips placing your hands on the seat of the chair directly under your shoulders. (See Figure 9.9, page 141.) Draw back through your hips as you extend forward through your spine to the crown of your head. Maintain the openness of your chest.

As you continue to pull back through the inner left thigh and shinbone, feel the stretch in your left calf and right hamstring. Breathe for thirty seconds working up to one minute. Bring your hands to your hips, inhale and press down through your legs and come up to a standing position. Change feet and repeat the sequence on the opposite side.

Classic Pose

Stand in Palm Tree Pose. Place your feet parallel, three and one half to four feet apart with your toes facing forward. Bring the palms of your hands together behind your back. Turn your fingers towards your spine and then up towards the ceiling in Namaste position. If you cannot comfortably hold this position, then cross your forearms behind our back, spreading your thumbs and index fingers around the creases at your opposite elbows.

Turn your left foot in approximately seventy-five degrees and your right foot out to ninety degrees. Turn your hips to the right so that your hips are parallel and your upper torso is facing your right leg. Inhale and lift your chest, bringing your side ribs up out of your pelvis. Spread your collar bone horizontally and draw your elbows back. (See Figure 9.10.)

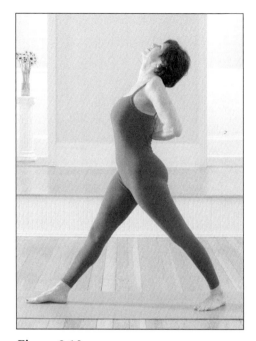

Figure 9.10
Spread your collarbone horizontally and draw your elbows back

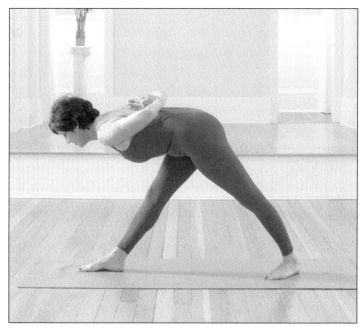

Figure 9.11
Draw back evenly through your hips as you extend forward
through your spine to the crown of your head

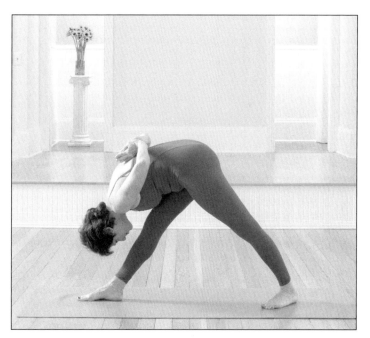

Figure 9.12
Extend your chest towards your right thigh as you move your
head towards your shin

Take your head back without straining your throat. Exhale and fold forward half way, drawing back evenly through your hips as you extend forward through your spine to the crown of your head. (See Figure 9.11, page 143.) Maintain the openness of your chest.

If you have flexibility in your hamstrings, on an exhalation, continue to fold from your hips down towards your right leg. (See Figure 9.12, page 143.) Extend your chest towards your right thigh as you move your head towards your shin. Remember to pull back through the inner left thigh and shinbone, feeling the stretch in your left calf and right hamstring. Breathe for twenty to thirty seconds working up to one minute. As you press down through your legs, inhale and extend through your spine to the crown of your head to come up to a standing position. Change feet and repeat the sequence on the opposite side.

Revolved Triangle
(Parivrtta Trikonasana)

We introduced you to Extended Triangle Pose (Utthita Trikonasana) in Chapter 6: Change Fat to Firm. You might have practiced this pose when you were working on strengthening and firming your legs and thighs. Now we will introduce you to a Revolved Triangle (Parivrtta Trikonasana). This is a more advanced standing pose. It involves twisting while maintaining your balance and stretching your hips and hamstrings. We will take you through this classic pose using a chair to make it more user friendly. We give you some options to complete the classic pose.

Preparation Pose with a Chair

Find a dining room or folding chair. Place the chair directly in front of you. Position your right foot between the front legs of the

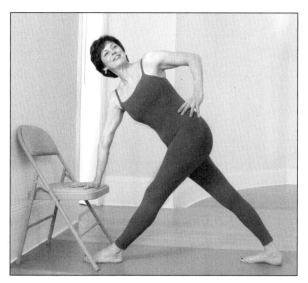

Figure 9.13
Twist towards your right as you bring your left ribs forward and your right shoulder towards the ceiling

chair and bring your left foot three and one half feet behind your the right foot. Line up your right heel and left heel with your left foot turned in seventy-five degrees. Place your hands on your hips and bring your left hip in line with your right hip.

Inhale and lift your chest, bringing your side ribs up out of your pelvis. Spread your collar bone horizontally and draw your elbows back. Exhale and fold forward from your hips placing your left hand on the seat of the chair directly in line with your big toe of your right foot. Place your right hand between your buttocks on your sacrum. Inhale and draw back through your hips as you extend forward through your spine to the crown of your head. Exhale and twist towards your right as you bring your left ribs forward and your right shoulder towards the ceiling. (See Figure 9.13.) Maintain an openness in your chest.

Option One

You can increase your stretch, moving closer to the classic pose, by lifting your right arm up and stretching through your fingers.

Option Two

If you have more flexibility in your hamstrings and hips, you may bring your left forearm down to the seat of the chair or place your left hand on a block at the little toe side of your right foot.

Breathe for twenty to thirty seconds working up to one minute. On an exhalation, press down through your legs, extend through your spine and come up and out of the twist, turning to the left. Change feet and repeat the sequence on the opposite side.

Revolved Right Angle Side Stretch (Parivrtta Parsvakonasana)

We introduced you to Right Angled Side Stretch (Utthita Parsvakonasana) in Chapter 6: Change Fat to Firm. You might have practiced this pose when you were working on strengthening and firming your legs and thighs. Now we will introduce you to Revolved Right Angled Side Stretch (Parivrtta Parsvakonasana). This is a more advanced standing pose. It involves twisting while maintaining your balance and stretching your hips and hamstrings. We will take you through this classic pose using a chair to make it more user friendly. We give you some options to complete the classic pose.

Preparation Pose One with a Chair

Find a dining room or folding chair. Place the chair at a wall and facing the chair, stand in Palm Tree Pose, approximately three feet away from the seat of the chair. Bend your right knee and place your right

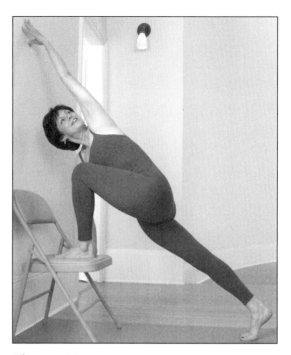

Figure 9.14
Stretch back through your left leg to your heel

foot on the seat of the chair. Bring your right knee directly over your right ankle and move your left foot slightly out to an eighty degree angle.

Place your hands on your hips and bring your left hip in line with your right hip.

Inhale and lift your chest, bringing your side ribs up out of your pelvis. Spread your collar bone horizontally and draw your elbows back. Exhale and fold forward from your hips placing your left hand on the seat of the chair on the big toe side of your right foot. Place your right hand between the buttocks at your sacrum.

Squeeze your hips together so that your right knee is in line with your right hip. Stretch actively back through your left leg through to your heel. Inhale and extend through your spine to the crown of your head. Exhale and twist towards your right as you bring your left ribs forward and your right shoulder towards the ceiling. Maintain an openness in your chest.

Inhale and stretch your right arm out to the side with your palm facing up towards the ceiling. With an exhalation, stretch your right arm towards your ear, creating a diagonal line from your right hip through to your fingertips. (See Figure 9.14, page 147.) Breathe for thirty seconds working up to one minute. Bring your right hand down to the little toe side of the right foot on the seat of the chair. Bring your right foot back to the floor and stand in Palm Tree Pose. Change feet and repeat the sequence on the opposite side.

Option One

If you want a deeper twist, cross your left upper arm over your right knee. Bring the palms of your hands together. On an exhalation, press your arm towards your thigh and your thigh towards your arm as you press your palms together. You can also slide your left hand down to hold the seat of the chair and stretch your right arm up next to your ear in a diagonal line.

Classic Pose

To complete the classic pose, eliminate the chair and place your front foot on the floor. You may use a block to support the hand that is reaching towards the floor. Repeat all of the above instructions.

Standing Hamstring and Adductor Stretch (Uttita Hasta Padangusthasana)

We introduced you to Standing Hamstring Stretch in Chapter 8: Stretch for Sports. You might have practiced this pose when you were stretching your hamstrings, quads and hips. The pose in Chapter 8 is the first part of Utthita Hasta Padangusthasana. Now you will learn the second part to complete this classic pose with a chair.

Preparation Pose with a Chair

Find a dining room or folding chair and place a blanket over the back of the chair. Stand in Palm Tree Pose, with the right side of your body facing the seat of the chair. Inhale and press down through your left leg. On an exhalation place your right foot on the blanket on the back of the chair. If you cannot place your foot that high, place your foot on a block that has been placed on the seat of the chair.

Bring your right thumb and index finger to the crease between your thigh and hip. Push down to level your hips. Inhale and extend through your spine. Exhale and fold sideways towards your right foot. Place your right hand at your shin or grab your big toe with your index and middle finger. Bring your right shoulder back to line up with your left shoulder and open your chest. Inhale and stretch your left arm out to the side with your palm facing up towards the ceiling. With an exhalation, stretch your left arm towards your ear, creating a diagonal line from your left heel through to your fingertips (See Figure 9.15.) Breathe for thirty seconds working up to one minute.

Press down through your left leg and release the pose to come up. Bring your right foot back to the floor in Palm Tree Pose. Repeat on the opposite side.

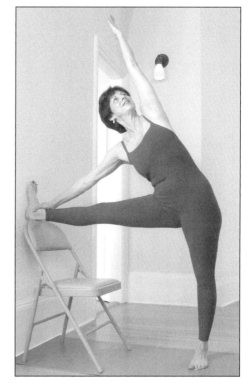

Figure 9.15
Bring your right shoulder back to line up with your left shoulder

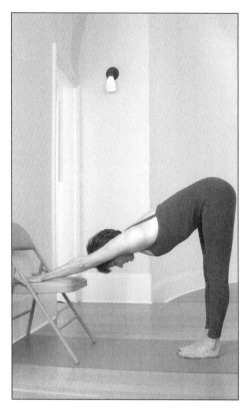

Figure 9.16
Pull your hips back, making your hips perpendicular to your ankles

Standing Forward Bend (Uttanasana)

We introduced you to Standing Forward Bend in Chapter 6: Change Fat to Firm. You might have practiced this pose when you were working on strengthening and firming your legs and thighs. Now you will learn to use a chair for a deeper stretch working towards the classic pose with your hands on the floor.

Pose with a Chair

Find a dining room or folding chair and place it at a wall. Stand three feet from the chair seat in Palm Tree Pose. Place your hands on your hips, inhale and lift your chest. Exhale and fold forward from your hips placing your hands on the seat of the chair. Reach from your bottom ribs forward, walking your fingertips forward. Continue to pull your hips back, making your hips perpendicular to your ankles. Feel the extension in your spine. (See Figure 9.16.) Breathe for thirty seconds building up to one minute. Release your hands and bring them to your hips. Inhale, lengthen your spine through the crown of your head. Exhale and press down through your legs to come up to Palm Tree Pose. Repeat on the opposite side.

Classic Pose

If you are more flexible in your hamstrings, and can continue to fold over from your hips, move your hands to the floor or to a block in front of your feet. Lift from your sitting bones and walk your hands back to line up your fingers with your toes. Remember to release your head and neck to allow the crown of your head to drop towards the floor.

✔ **Elise's Note:** If your hamstrings are extremely tight, you may place your feet hip-width apart as you do this pose.

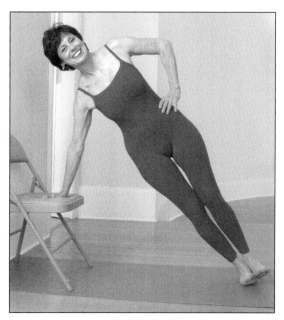

Figure 9.17
Bring your right shoulder directly over your right hand

Arm Balance and Back Strengthener
(Vasisthasana)

This pose strengthens your arms, back muscles and side body.

Pose with a Chair

Find a dining room or folding chair and place it at a wall. Stand two feet from the chair with your right side facing the seat in Palm Tree Pose. Place your right hand on the seat of the chair. Walk your feet out from the chair so that your weight is on the outer side of your right foot. Bring your left foot in line with your right foot so that your left foot is resting on your right instep. Bring your right shoulder directly over your right hand. Inhale and stretch your left arm up as you find the alignment of Tadasana as your body is leaning to the right side forming a diagonal line. (See Figure 9.17.) Breathe for twenty seconds working up to one minute.

Bring your left hand down to the seat of the chair and place your feet to face the chair. Stretch your arms forward towards the back of the chair to feel the stretch in your back. Place your hands of your hips, inhale and come up to a standing position. Now turn to the opposite side and repeat the sequence.

Classic Pose

We introduced you to Downward Facing Dog, Adho Mukha Svanasana, in Chapter 10. To begin this classic pose, you need to start in Downward Facing Dog. Now, Turn to your right side so that the little toe side of your right foot is pressing into the floor in line with your right hand. Bring your left foot in line with your right foot so that your left foot is resting on your right instep. Inhale and stretch your left arm up as you find the alignment of Tadasana as your body is leaning to the right side forming a diagonal line. Be sure to lift your outer right thigh up towards the ceiling and keep your head in line with your sternum. (See Figure 9.18, page 153.) Breathe for twenty seconds working up to one minute.

Inhale and on an exhalation, bring your right hand down to the floor returning to Downward Facing Dog. Repeat the sequence on the opposite side.

Option One

If cannot find your balance or your arms are not strong enough to create the correct alignment, your may place your left foot on the floor, in front of your body to create more stability and the correct alignment to be able to open your chest. (See Figure 9.19, page 153.) This is a way to build your strength to work up to the classic pose.

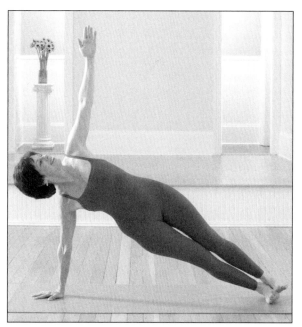

Figure 9.18
Find the alignment of Tadasana as your body is
leaning to the right side forming a diagonal line

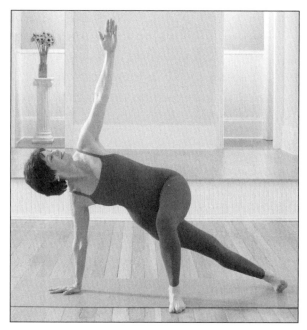

Figure 9.19
Place your left foot on the floor, in front of your body
to create more stability and the correct alignment

Camel Pose
(Ustrasana)

This classic pose stretches your thighs and opens your solar plexus, chest, and heart. It teaches you to lift your thoracic spine up and out of your lower back improving flexibility in your entire back. Using a chair will help you to learn how to lift your mid-back out of your lower back, reducing lower back pain.

Pose with a Chair

Find a folding chair and place it at a wall. Kneel with your back to the chair and your feet under the seat of the chair so that your buttocks are three inches from the edge of the seat of the chair. Place your hands on your hips, inhale and lift your chest up out of your lower back. Keeping your lift, exhale and place your hands back on the seat of the chair and continue to lift feeling the arch in your mid-back. If you have more flexibility, you may walk your hands down the front legs of the folding chair for a deeper stretch. Press your tailbone towards your pubis, stretching the fronts of your thighs and align your hips over your knees. Continue to breathe and extend the crown of your head back. (See Figure 9.20.) Breathe for twenty seconds working up to one minute.

Classic Pose

As you increase in flexibility, remove the chair and use two blocks by the sides of your ankles to support your hands. The classic pose is achieved when you can place your hands on your heels.

✔ **Elise's Note:** Backbends are most beneficial when you repeat the pose at least two times during a practice.

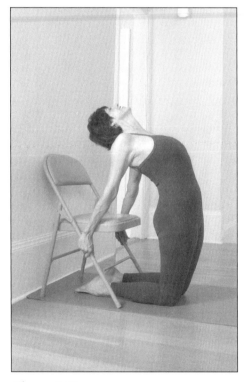

Figure 9.20
Stretch the fronts of your thighs and align your hips over your knees

Chair Twist
(Chair Bharadvajasana)

We introduced you to a similar twist in Chapter 3: Stretch In the Office. (See Figure 3.12, page 32.) This classic pose is a safe and deeper twist for all back conditions. This theraputic pose focuses on twisting from your lower ribs through to the crown of your head. You can maintain the natural curve of your lower back for the safest position.

Pose with Chair

Find a folding chair and place it at a wall. Sit on the chair so that your right thigh is facing the back of the chair. Place a block between your thighs and bring your feet parallel. Place your hands on the back of the chair. Inhale and lift your spine, bringing your lower back into its natural concave curve. Exhale and press the right palm into the back of the chair and twist your body from your left waist towards the right.

To deepen the twist, pull with your left hand while you are pushing with your right hand. Square your shoulders, feeling your shoulder blades flatten on your back, and allow your neck and head to follow the twist of your spine. Drop your shoulders from your ears and be sure to extend through your upper arms to your elbows slightly out to your sides. (See Figure 9.21.) Breathe for thirty seconds working up to one minute.

Inhale and lift up through your spine. Exhale and release your hands to come out of the twist. Turn to the other side and repeat the sequence.

✔ **Elise's Note:** Twists are most beneficial when you repeat the pose at least two times in a practice.

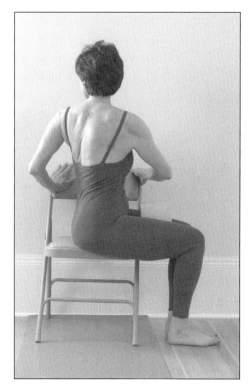

Figure 9.21
Square your shoulders, feeling your shoulder blades flatten on your back

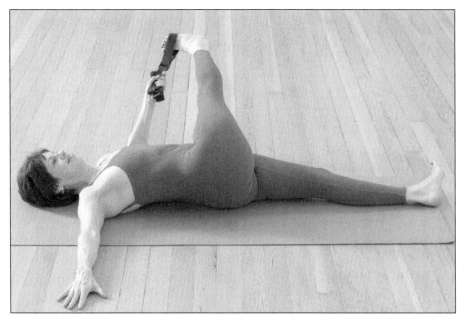

Figure 9.22
Feel the twist as you anchor your right foot to the floor

Spinal Twist and Hip Opener (One-legged Jathara Parivartanasana)

We introduced you to a floor twist with knees bent (Jathara Parivartanasana) in Chapter 6: Change Fat to Firm. Now we show you a variation that focuses on the hips and hamstrings for a deeper stretch.

Pose with a Strap

Lie down on your back, bend your right knee, bringing your leg towards your chest as you place a strap around the ball of your right foot. Place a blanket under your head if your chin is higher than your forehead.

Keeping your left leg firmly on the floor, lift your right leg towards the ceiling. Breathe for five breaths. Hold the strap with your left hand and place your right hand out to the side in line with your right shoulder, palm facing down. Inhale and extend through both legs. Exhale and roll on to the left side of your hip bringing your right hip towards the ceiling. Turn your left foot towards the left so that your little toe touches the floor. Bring your sacrum perpendicular to the floor.

To lengthen your right hip from your waist, place your thumb and index finger in the crease of your right leg and push towards your left foot. Bring your right hand back to the floor and feel the twist as you anchor your right shoulder to the floor. (See Figure 9.22, page 156.) Breathe for thirty seconds working up to one minute.

Inhale and on an exhalation, swing your right leg back up towards the ceiling and bring your back flat on the floor. Release the strap and slowly bring your right leg down to the floor, extending through your heel and the ball of your foot. Repeat the sequence on the opposite side.

Classic Pose

As your legs become more flexible, you can hold the outer side of your right foot with your left hand to practice a more classic version of this pose. Then repeat holding your left foot with your right hand.

Classic Yoga Relaxation

Lie down in Savasana. Find your alignment in Tadasana on the floor. Let go equally with your legs and arms, palms of your hands facing up. Feel your head centered, neither rolling to the right or the left. Allow

Sthira sukham asanam
(Find the steadiness and the ease.)
— Yoga Sutra 2.46 from Patanjali

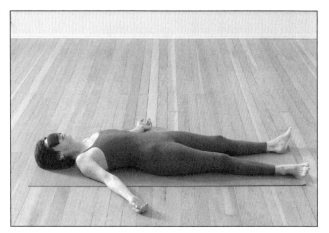

Figure 9.23
Let go equally with your legs and arms, palms of your hands facing up

your eyes to relax downward with your jaw and tongue relaxed. (See Figure 9.23.)

Drop down into the earth, feeling the support as you observe the lightness and openness of your front body. Observe the evenness of your breath as you continue to inhale and exhale. Feel the steadiness and the ease of the moment. The true nature of yoga is the balance of the all opposites, light and dark, up and down, in and out. You continue to observe your place in the universe as you continue to seek balance in all aspects of your life. This is an opportunity to find your special place in all life experiences.

When you are ready, take a deep breath, gently move your fingers and toes, roll to your right side and press into the floor with your left palm to come up to a sitting position.

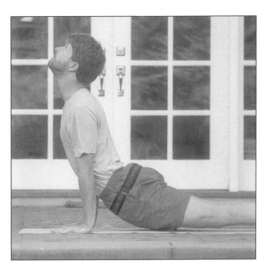

chapter 10

Energize the Whole Body

Do you ever feel . . .

. . . your energy is playing hide and seek with you? You have a hard time getting out of bed in the morning or your brain has a regular appointment with an afternoon slump. Even though you know it would be good to exercise, you just don't have the energy to get up and do it.

Here are some stretches that you can do immediately upon arising or when you need an energy boost to revitalize you. Your energy is always available to you. With the right tools, you can access it when you need it. The poses are planned to energize the body and stimulate clearer thinking. And it's better for you than coffee and completely organic!

✔ **Equipment Note:** A yoga sticky mat (if you're on a slippery surface or rug), two to three blankets, and a chair.

Breathing

This stretch becomes a swinging motion to increase your energy.

> Stand with your feet parallel, hip-width apart, with your hips over your heels and your arms down by your sides.
>
> To start the swinging motion, inhale as you bring your arms behind you and up over your head in a circular motion.
>
> Continue to swing your arms, exhale, and bring your arms down in front of you along the outside of your thighs as you bend forward from your hips. Let your arms continue back until they reach hip level, parallel to the floor. Let your head hang down.
>
> Now swing your arms forward and inhale, stretching your arms forward and up over your head, bringing the upper torso along with them to a standing position.
>
> Exhale and continue to bring the arms around to the back in a circular motion until the hands come down by your sides.
>
> Repeat this sequence at least ten times.

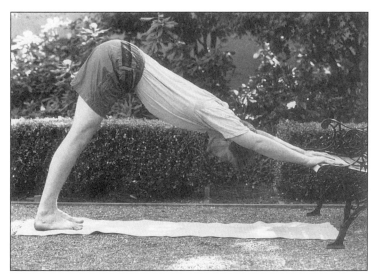

Figure 10.1
Walk back far enough to keep your buttocks lifted and your lower back in its natural curve

Remember to breathe in rhythm with the movements, keeping your knees slightly bent to create fluid motions.

Stretching

Downward Facing Dog (*Adho Mukha Svanasana*)

Find a dining room-style chair, a folding chair, or a bench and place the heels of the hands on the front edge of the seat.

Walk your feet back far enough so that you are bending from the hips and your buttocks are lifted toward the ceiling, with your lower back in its natural curve. Your feet should be back farther than your hips. (See Figure 10.1.)

Press down through your palms, particularly through the knuckles at the base of your index and middle fingers. Stretch up through your arms, spine, and pelvis to your buttocks bones as you stretch back through your legs. Release your neck and head.

Breathe and hold for thirty seconds, building up to one minute. Be sure to bring your shoulder blades toward your chest and keep the lower back in its natural concave curve. If this is not possible, bend your knees, tilt your tailbone up, moving the shoulder blades toward your chest, bringing your lower back into its natural curve. As you practice, you will be able to slowly straighten your knees, keeping the alignment of your spine.

On an exhalation, walk the feet toward the chair. Inhale and release your hands.

Stand firmly on the floor, stretching your arms out to your sides and over your head. Then exhale and bring your arms down by your sides.

Variation

This is the real Dog Pose and it requires more flexible hips, shoulders, and hamstring muscles. Use a yoga sticky mat if the surface is slippery.

Lie on your abdomen with your palms flat on the floor under your shoulders, spreading your fingers out equally. Be sure that your middle fingers are facing directly forward. Your fingertips should be at the edge of your shoulders.

Inhale, exhale, and press down with your palms, lifting your body so that you are on your hands and knees. Curl your toes under so that you are on the balls of your feet.

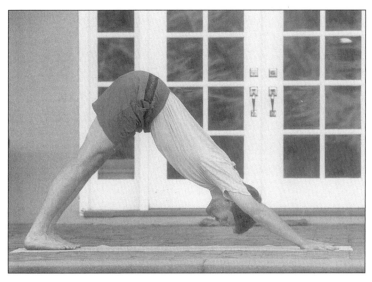

Figure 10.2
The real Downward Facing Dog, requiring more flexibility in the hips, shoulders, and hamstrings

Bring the lower back into its natural concave curve, with the buttocks bones lifting to the ceiling.

Inhale and exhale, pressing down through the palms, and lift from the tailbone, bringing the knees off of the floor. Stretch up through your arms, spine, and pelvis to your buttocks bones as you stretch back through your legs and bring your shoulder blades toward your chest. Release your neck and head. (See Figure 10.2.)

Breathe and hold for thirty seconds, building up to one minute. Keep the lower back in its natural concave curve. If this is difficult, bend your knees slightly, slowly straightening as you become more flexible.

To relax, bring your knees down to the floor, bring the tops of your feet to the floor and slowly stretch the buttocks back to the heels. Bring the arms down by your sides and relax into Child's Pose. (See page 53 and Figure 8.14, page 119.)

✔ **Elise's Note:** Dogs have found over the centuries that this pose is very beneficial. It stretches the spine, opens the chest, brings circulation into the brain, and stretches the hamstrings. It is specifically given as a therapeutic pose for fatigue. What more could you want?

✔ **Carol's Note:** If you are stranded on a desert island, this is the pose you want to do. It does everything for you and it really feels good.

Upward Facing Dog (Urdhva Mukha Svanasana)

Find a dining room-style chair, a folding chair, or a bench and place the heels of the hands on the front edge of the seat. Walk your feet back far enough, with your palms flat on the chair and your hands directly under your shoulders, spreading your fingers out equally. Be sure that your middle fingers are facing directly forward.

Drop your pelvis down, coming onto the balls of your feet. The heels of your hands should be in line with your lower ribs. (See Figure 10.3, page 165.)

Inhale and press the palms into the chair, lifting the upper body, feeling the lift from the pelvis through the crown of the head.

Turn the upper arms out to draw the shoulder blades in toward the back ribs to open the chest.

Exhale, firming the buttocks and legs, keeping the stretch back through the heels. Extend through the crown of the head and you may bring the head back, being careful to not compress the vertebrae of the neck.

Breathe and hold for thirty seconds, building to one minute.

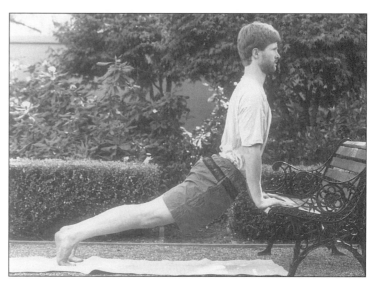

Figure 10.3
Drop your pelvis down, pressing the palms into the chair, lifting the upper body

Pressing your palms down, bring your buttocks back over your heels. On an exhalation, walk the feet toward the chair. Inhale and release your hands.

Stand firmly on the floor, stretching your arms out to your sides and over your head. Then exhale and bring your arms down by your sides.

Variation

This is the real Upward Facing Dog, which is a deeper backward bend that strengthens the back. Use a yoga sticky mat if needed.

Lie on your abdomen, with your palms flat on the floor under your shoulders, spreading your fingers out equally. Be sure that your middle fingers are facing directly forward. The heels of your hands are in line with your lower ribs, and the middle of your hands are in line with your breastbone.

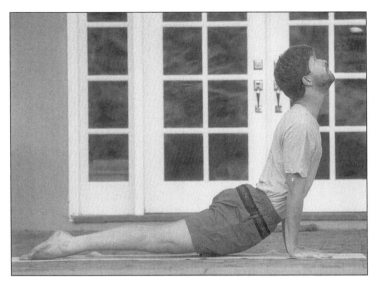

Figure 10.4
The real Upward Facing Dog—a deeper backward bend

Bring the tops of the feet onto the floor. Inhale and squeeze the buttocks.

Exhale and press your palms and tops of the feet into the floor, lifting the legs and the upper body. You should feel the lift from the pelvis through the crown of your head. (See Figure 10.4.) If you cannot raise your legs off the floor and feel a lift of your spine, curl the toes under with the balls of the feet on the floor, and press down into the floor to lift your legs.

This is the completed position of Upward Facing Dog. Now with an exhalation, drop your knees down, bend your elbows, and bring your chest down to the floor to relax.

✔ **Elise's Note:** This is a backward bend where the arms and legs are strengthened to allow the chest to open. It is excellent for rounded shoulders and kyphosis (extreme rounded mid-back), and a great complement to Downward Facing Dog. With the chair poses, you may move from

Downward Dog to Upward Dog in one fluid motion, repeating several times to energize and loosen the spine.

Sun Salutation (Surya Namaskar)

This is a flowing movement of twelve postures to limber and stretch all the muscles of the body. The series is meant to be done in one continuous movement. In the beginning, you may need to focus on each posture individually. Use a yoga sticky mat if needed.

All the instructions are listed first so that you can get a feel for the movements. Then see pages 170–173 for a pictorial view of the movement series. (You may want to record the instructions on an audio tape to listen to as you follow the photos.)

Stand in Palm Tree Pose (see Figure 2.8, page 18), with your feet together and your head, shoulders, and hips in line with your heels.

Inhale, and on exhalation, bring the palms of the hands together, with your thumbs touching your breastbone. This is a traditional greeting in India. (See Figure 10.5, page 170.)

Inhale and stretch your arms out in front, lifting them overhead so that your arms line up with your head, shoulders, hips, and heels. (See Figure 10.6, page 170.)

Exhale and bend forward from the hips, bringing your arms out in front. (See Figure 10.7, page 170.) If this strains your back, bring your arms out to your sides as you bend.

Continue down toward the floor with your fingertips in line with your toes. If your hands do not touch the floor, let your fingers dangle. Inhale and extend your spine. Exhale and bring your palms toward the floor by the sides of your feet. (See Figure 10.8, page 170.)

If your back is rounded, bend your knees slightly to bend from your hips, taking the strain off your back.

Bring the right leg back, with the knee on the floor and the top of the foot resting on the floor. Your left knee should line up with your left ankle bone. Drop your right thigh toward the floor, stretching the right front thigh into a lunge, with the knee now coming slightly in front of the ankle.

Exhale and curl the toes of your right foot under, bringing the ball of the foot on the floor. (See Figure 10.9, page 171.) As you become more confident, you may lift the arms over your head while in the lunge position, stretching your spine and opening your chest.

Inhale and bring the left leg back to join the right leg. Your body should now be in a straight line, with the palms directly under the shoulders. (See Figure 10.10, page 171.)

Exhale and bring the knees, chest, and chin down to the floor, with the buttocks slightly lifted. (See Figure 10.11, page 171.)

Inhale and drop your pelvis, pressing the palms down, and lift your head and upper torso while lifting your legs off the floor. Lift up into Upward Facing Dog. (See Figure 10.12, page 172.)

Exhale and lift the pelvis while pressing the palms into the floor, and stretch backward through the legs into Downward Facing Dog. (See Figure 10.13, page 172.)

Inhale and hop to bring your right foot forward, placing it between the palms of your hands and stretching into another lunge. (See Figure 10.14, page 172.)

If you cannot place the right foot between the palms during the hop, drop the left knee to the floor and grab your right ankle with your right hand to move it forward.

Stretch your left thigh down toward the floor, lunging your right knee forward. You may lift the arms over your head while in the lunge position, stretching your spine and opening your chest.

Exhale and bring the left foot forward to line up with the right foot, dropping your head and straightening your legs into a forward bend. (See Figure 10.15, page 173.)

Inhale and stretch the arms out in front and over your head as your bring your upper body to a standing position. (See Figures 10.16 and 10.17, page 173.) If this strains your back, bring your arms out to the sides as you come up to a standing position.

Exhale and bring the palms together to the greeting position at the chest. (See Figure 10.18, page 173.)

Slowly bring your arms back to your sides into Palm Tree Pose.

Repeat this whole series at least three times, creating more of a fluid movement as you learn the sequence.

✔ **Elise's Note:** This is a traditional sequence that has been done by Indians at sunrise for over 2,000 years to wake up the body and mind. *Surya* means sun and *Namaskar* means greetings or salutations.

✔ **Carol's Note:** Elise had a student who only practiced the Sun Salutation for fifteen years. He remained very limber with only this one routine. This stretch is beautiful to watch and feels wonderful to learn.

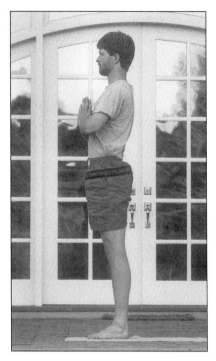

Figure 10.5
In Palm Tree Pose, bring your palms together with your thumbs touching your breastbone

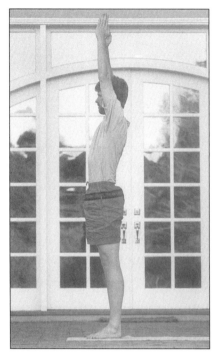

Figure 10.6
Lift the arms overhead, keeping them in line with your head, shoulders, hips, and heels

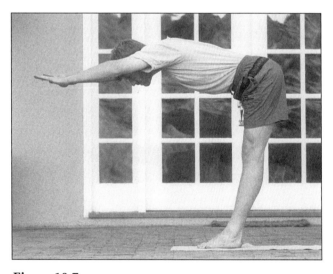

Figure 10.7
Exhale and bend forward from the hips, bringing your arms out in front

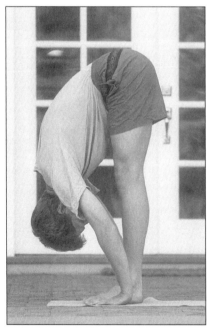

Figure 10.8
Inhale as you bring your palms toward the floor by the sides of your feet

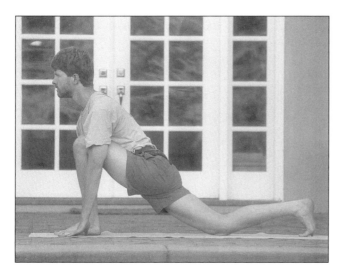

Figure 10.9
Drop your right thigh toward the floor, stretching into a lunge, curling the toes under

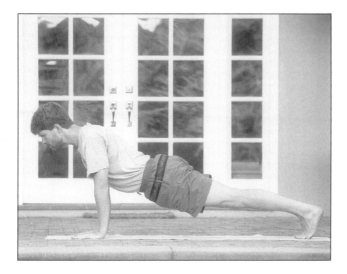

Figure 10.10
Bringing the left leg back, your body should now be in a straight line

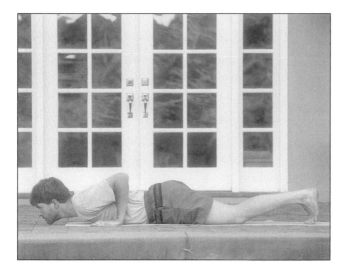

Figure 10.11
Exhale and bring the knees, chest, and chin down to the floor with the buttocks slightly lifted

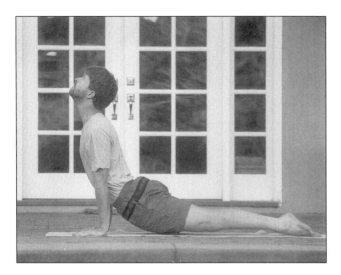

Figure 10.12
Drop your pelvis, press the palms down and lift your head and upper torso while lifting your legs off the floor into Upward Facing Dog

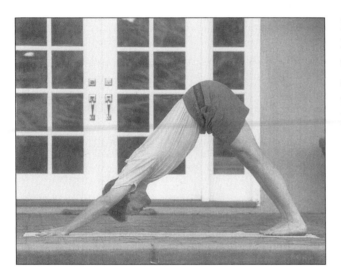

Figure 10.13
Lift the pelvis while pressing the palms into the floor, and stretch backward through the legs into Downward Facing Dog

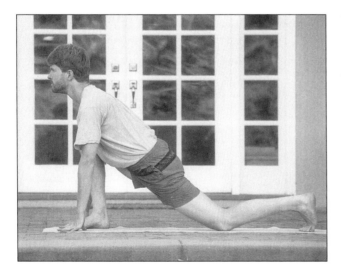

Figure 10.14
Stretch into another lunge, dropping the left thigh toward the floor

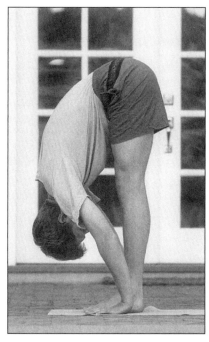

Figure 10.15
Straighten into a forward bend

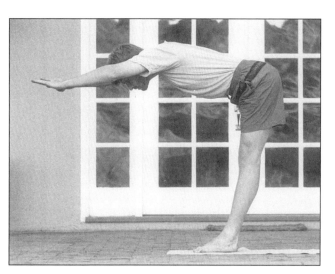

Figure 10.16
Inhale and stretch your arms out in front

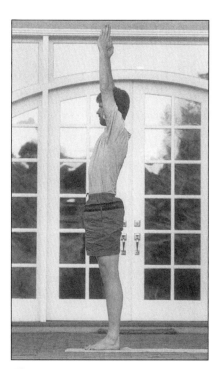

Figure 10.17
Bring your arms overhead as you raise your upper body

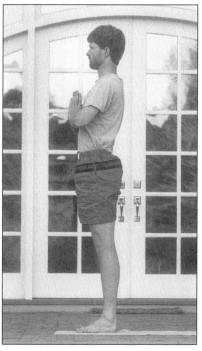

Figure 10.18
Exhale and bring the palms together

Bridging on Wall to Shoulder Stand (Setu Bandha and Salamba Sarvangasana)

Get two blankets and fold them into a primary fold. (For folding instructions, see Figure 12.1, page 200.) Use three blankets if your neck and shoulders are tight. Place the blankets near the wall.

Lie down on your back on the blanket so that your buttocks are at the wall and your shoulders are a couple of inches from the far edge of the blanket. Be sure that your shoulders are at the folded end of the blanket.

Stretch your legs up the wall and extend through your heels. Bring your arms down by your sides, placing your palms down on the floor. Bend your knees and slide your feet down until the bottoms of your feet are flat on the wall, parallel and hip-width apart. Your legs will be at a right angle.

Inhale and exhale, pressing the feet into the wall, lifting the buttocks and back off the floor until you come onto the tops of your shoulders at the edge of the blanket. Interlace your fingers behind your back, with your palms facing your back. (See Figure 10.19, page 175.)

Stretch through your arms, bringing your little fingers down to the floor.

Release your fingers, keeping your elbows in line with your shoulders, and place your palms on your back. Walk your feet up to knee height, forming a right angle. Breathe and continue to move your buttocks away from the wall and your shoulder blades toward your chest. This opens your chest and aligns your body.

Breathe and hold for thirty seconds, building up to one minute.

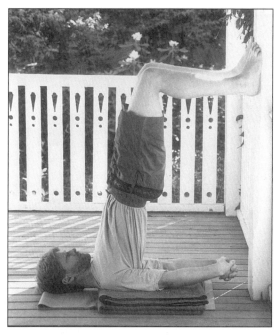

Figure 10.19
Pressing your feet into the wall, lift your buttocks and back off the floor until you're on the tops of your shoulders

To come out of this pose: Inhale and stretch your arms over your head. Exhale and slowly roll the spine down to the floor, vertebra by vertebra. Gently roll your shoulders over the edge of the blanket, placing your shoulders on the floor and your lower back on the blanket.

Placing your arms at shoulder height, bend your elbows at a right angle with your palms facing the ceiling. Let your legs rest on the wall. Breathe and rest for one minute.

Bring your knees to your chest, roll to your side, and use your hands to bring your upper body to an upright position.

✔ **Elise's Note:** Take your time with each of the following variations and build up consistently. A suggestion is to do each variation for a minute for a week before doing the next variation. This will prevent overstretching the neck.

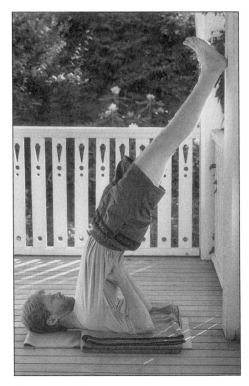

Figure 10.20
To come out of the pose, walk your feet up the wall until your legs are straight

Variation One

Starting with Bridging on Wall pose (legs at a right angle on the wall), walk your feet all the way up the wall until your legs are straight. Rest on your heels, with the bottoms of your feet stretching off the wall. (See Figure 10.20.)

Breathe and hold for thirty seconds, building up to one minute. This is preparation for Shoulder Stand (Variation Three).

Release your hands and slowly roll your spine onto the floor, letting your heels slide down.

Variation Two

Starting with Bridging on Wall pose (legs at a right angle with feet flat on the wall), inhale and lift your left leg off of the wall, stretching from your pelvis through the heel. (See Figure 10.21, page 177.)

Align your shoulders, hips, and left heel. Place your left foot back on the wall and lift your right leg, stretching through the heel.

Bring both feet flat on the wall, legs at a right angle. Release your hands and slowly roll your spine onto the floor, letting your heels slide down.

Variation Three: Shoulder Stand

Starting with Bridging on Wall pose (legs at a right angle with feet flat on the wall), inhale and lift your left leg off the wall and then lift your right leg off the wall to balance in a shoulder stand. Lift up from your pelvis through your heels, aligning your shoulders, hips, and legs. (See Figure 10.22, page 177.)

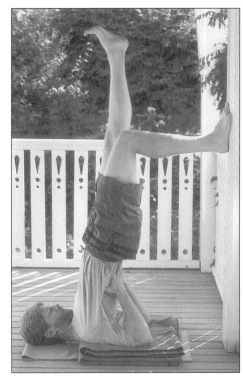

Figure 10.21
Inhale and lift your left leg off of the wall, stretching from your pelvis through the heel

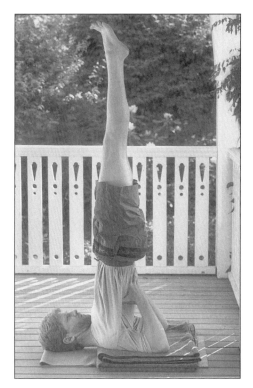

Figure 10.22
Lift both legs off the wall to balance in a shoulder stand

✔ **Elise's Note:** The most important point is to go slowly, with no jerky or sloppy movements.

Bridging on Wall pose is wonderful for opening the chest and loosening the shoulders. Shoulder Stand is an inversion that stimulates the glandular system as well as takes the weight off of your legs, especially if you've been standing on them all day. This is also a great energizer if you have to keep going into the evening!

Relaxation *(Savasana)*

You may record this on audio tape.

Lie on your back, with your arms to your sides, legs straight and relaxed, and your head in the center. Take three deep breaths and begin to imagine that each inhalation brings you new energy and vitality. With each exhalation, you feel the release of tension throughout your body.

Bring your breath into your feet and your legs, feeling the energy flow through each cell in the lower part of your body. Exhale and feel any tension and stress release through each cell of your lower body.

Now feel the breath move up into the thighs, buttocks, pelvis, and lower back. Exhale and feel all of the tension releasing.

Bring your breath into your spine and back muscles. Feel the energy flowing through the vertebrae, creating space and alignment. Exhale and let go of any tension in this area.

Inhale and feel the breath move into your belly, chest, and shoulders, moving all the way down to your arms and through your fingertips. Exhale and release all of the tension that remains in your upper body.

Inhale and breathe into your throat, neck, face, and skull. Exhale and feel your brain relax as the face muscles soften into total relaxation. Feel a balance between aliveness and total relaxation.

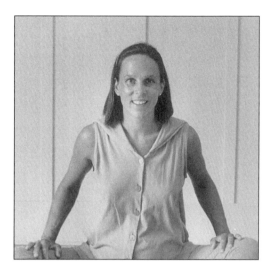

chapter 11

Harmonize Your Hormones

Menstrual Cycle Relief, Pregnancy, Healthy Menopause

Do you ever feel . . .

. . . your female hormones are playing havoc with you? And you just can't seem to get a grip on yourself? Whether you have cramps, or are having a baby, or are about to move into a new phase of your female life, you want relief from the discomfort and to regain a sense of control over your emotions.

Here are some poses to remedy your situation. These stretches help with menstrual disorders, the birthing process, and the physical effects of menopause. No matter what stage of life you are experiencing, yoga stretches also calm the mind and soothe the emotional responses that accompany hormonal changes.

For some of the following poses, you'll need some blankets folded in specific ways. Use the blanket chart that illustrates how to do three basic folds: primary, double, and triple. (See Figure 12.1, page 200.) The folds progress from a primary to a double or a triple fold. The type of fold or folds required for a pose will be indicated at the beginning of the instructions.

✔ **Equipment Note:** A yoga sticky mat, three blankets, a towel, a book or yoga block, a yoga belt, and a yoga bolster or a large, rectangular sofa pillow.

Breathing

This exercise is appropriate for all three conditions.

Get three blankets and one towel. Fold one blanket into a triple fold. (See Figure 12.1, page 200.) Fold the other two blankets into squares.

Sit down so that the long blanket (triple fold) is behind you, place a blanket square on each side of your thighs, and place a towel where you will place your head.

Bend your knees so that the soles of your feet come together, forming a diamond shape with your legs. Drop your knees so the outer sides of your thighs and calves lie on the folded blanket squares. If you have tight inner thighs and your legs do not touch the blankets, fold the blankets again to make them higher or get additional blankets or pillows.

Lay your spine down lengthwise on top of the long folded blanket, placing the back of your head on the towel, so that you can drop your chin toward your chest.

Let your arms drop down at a forty-five degree angle away from your body. Let your shoulders fall away from the blanket and let your legs relax.

Inhale, bringing the breath down into the belly, filling it like a balloon. Feel your diaphragm muscles move down toward the base of your pelvis. Feel it spreading from the navel to the side of your waist.

Exhale and feel the balloon slowly release the air, letting the diaphragm relax and soften.

Repeat this conscious breathing ten times. Allow all of your reproductive organs and entire lower pelvic region to relax.

Stretching

Menstrual Cycle Relief

Reclined Hero (*Supta Virasana*)

Get a yoga bolster or a rectangular sofa pillow and a book or yoga block. Then take two blankets and fold each into a triple fold.

Place the block or book next to the short edge of one blanket at the end of the bolster or pillow. Place the second blanket on top of the first so that the end of the top blanket is approximately six inches from the short edge where the block is placed.

This allows the other end of the top blanket to be folded over to make a pillow for your head and to prevent your lumbar spine from becoming too concave.

Kneel over the block, with your knees hip-width apart. Sit back so that your buttocks rest on the block and your heels are to the sides of your buttocks, with the tops of your feet on the floor. Be sure that your toes are pointing backward. (This is Virasana.)

Place your hands behind your feet and lift your buttocks, tucking them under, and slowly roll your spine down to lie on the folded blankets. Be sure that the edge of the top blanket is in line with the bottom ribs.

Stretch your arms over your head, interlacing your fingers, with your palms facing away from your head. Inhale and stretch the upper torso away from the pelvis as you lengthen from your thighs to your knees.

Exhale and let your arms relax at your sides, palms facing up. (See Figure 11.1, page 183.)

Breathe and hold for two minutes, building up to five minutes.

Relax and feel a gentle stretch in your thighs. Continue breathing into your lower pelvic region.

Bring your hands to the sides and press your palms down into the floor to lift your chest and upper torso off of the support. Come forward into Child's Pose and relax. (See page 53 and Figure 8.14, page 125.)

✔ **Elise's Note:** This pose stretches the reproductive organs, relaxes the lower pelvic region, and helps to reduce menstrual cramping. If you want more of a stretch, decrease the height of the

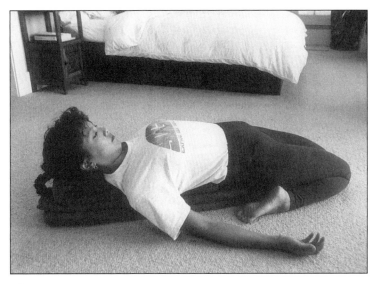

Figure 11.1
As you lie on the blankets/bolster, stretch the upper torso away from the pelvis and relax your arms at your sides

support behind you. If it's too low and a strain on your back, build up the height with more blankets until it's comfortable. Another reclined pose that helps to relieve menstrual cramping is Reclined Bound Angle Pose. (See Figure 12.9, page 211.)

✔ **Carol's Note:** It's worth taking the time to fold the blankets and enjoy the stretch.

Head to Knee Pose (*Janusirsasana*)

Sit on the floor with your legs together, stretched out in front of you. Bring your hands to your right buttock and move the flesh and skin out of the way so that you are sitting on your "sitting bones." Repeat on the left side.

If your lower back is rounded, sit on the edge of a folded blanket to help you correctly position your lower back.

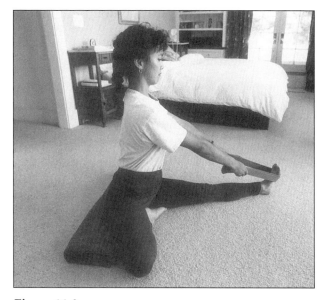

Figure 11.2
Place a belt on the ball of your foot and with an inhalation, lift your spine up

Bring the arms down by your sides and lifting up through your spine, stretch out through your heels, pressing your thighs to the floor. This is Staff or Rod Pose. (See Figure 8.9, page 119.)

Bend the right knee to the side so that your heel is near your right groin. Turn the upper torso so that your chest faces over the center of your left leg. Place a belt on the ball of your left foot. With an inhalation, lift your spine up. (See Figure 11.2.)

Exhale and bend from your hips, stretching forward over your left leg. Be sure to keep your chest open and your lower back concave. Keep your left leg straight and your shoulders relaxed.

Breathe and hold for one minute.

Now to relax completely into the pose, place a blanket or bolster on your left leg and let your forehead rest on this support.

Release the belt and relax your arms to the sides, palms facing up.

Breathe and hold for one minute, building up to two minutes. Totally relax your belly and the lower pelvic area.

Slowly inhale and lift your upper torso back into a sitting position. Stretch your right leg back out and repeat on the opposite side.

This pose relaxes the reproductive organs and relieves cramping.

Full Forward Bend
(Paschimottanasana)

Sit on the floor with your legs together, stretched out in front of you. Make sure that you are sitting on your "sitting bones."

If your lower back is rounded, sit on the edge of a folded blanket to help you correctly position your lower back.

Bring the arms down by your sides and lifting up through your spine, stretch out through your heels, pressing your thighs to the floor. This is Staff or Rod Pose. (See Figure 8.9, page 119.)

Inhale and lift your arms over your head, with your palms facing each other. Breathe and feel the stretch up through your spine, lifting the upper torso from your pelvis.

Turn the palms to face forward and with an exhalation, bend at the hips, bringing the upper torso and arms forward, holding a belt around the balls of your feet. (See Figure 11.3, page 186.) Keep your chest open and your lower back concave. Make sure your legs are straight and your shoulders relaxed.

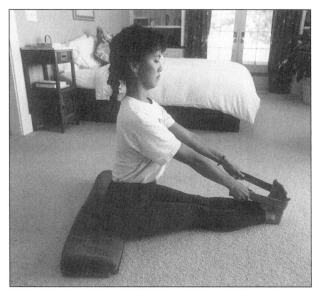

Figure 11.3
With an exhalation, bend at the hips, bringing the upper torso and arms forward while holding a belt around the balls of your feet

Breathe and hold for one minute.

Now to relax completely into the pose, place a blanket or a bolster on your legs and let your forehead rest on this support. Release the belt and relax your arms to the sides, palms facing up.

Breathe and hold for one minute, building up to two minutes. Totally relax your belly and the lower pelvic area.

Slowly inhale and lift your upper torso back into a sitting position.

This is a very powerful pose that calms the nervous system as well as relaxes the reproductive organs and decreases cramping. As you practice this, you can build up to five minutes in the pose, which will give you even stronger benefits.

Pregnancy

In this next section are some poses that are especially helpful during pregnancy. In addition, below are some suggested poses that you will find in the other sections of the book. Choose the ones you feel are best suited for you. We have listed them in the order we think is the best progression:

- Cat Cow—see pages 52–53 in Chapter 5
- Any postures from Chapter 6
- Downward Facing Dog—see pages 161– 164 in Chapter 10, but do with feet placed eighteen inches apart
- Wide-Angled Standing Pose—see pages 115–116 in Chapter 8

Bound Angle Pose with Legs on the Wall (*Baddha Konasana*)

To get into this position, sit with the right side of your body next to the wall. Have your knees bent, with your feet on the floor. Now lean back and swing your legs up the wall, bringing your back to the floor. Make sure the buttocks are on the floor.

With an exhalation, bend the knees and slide the feet down the wall, bringing the soles of the feet together and the knees to the sides.

Inhale, pressing your heels in toward each other. Exhale, placing your hands on your thighs, and press your thighs toward the wall. (See Figure 11.4, page 188.)

Breathe and hold for one minute.

Now relax your arms onto the floor out to the sides with your palms facing up.

Breathe and relax your entire pelvic area for four minutes.

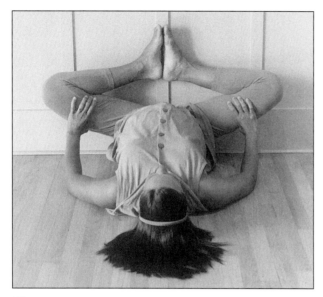

Figure 11.4
Press your heels toward each other while pressing
your thighs toward the wall

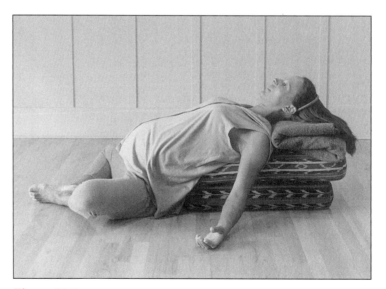

Figure 11.5
If you have difficulty lying on your back or feel extremely
tired, do Reclined Bound Angle Pose

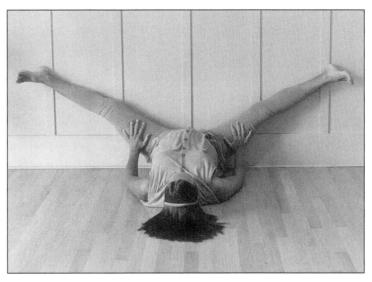

Figure 11.6
Stretch your legs out to the sides as far as possible, placing your hands on your thighs to keep the legs straight

Stretch the legs back up on the wall, straightening them. This position leads into the next pose.

If you have difficulty lying on your back during the last few months of pregnancy, do Bound Angle Pose. (See Figure 8.11, page 121.) If you feel extremely tired, do Reclined Bound Angle Pose. (See Figure 11.5, page 188 and also Figure 12.9, page 211.)

Wide-Angled Pose on the Wall
(Upavistha Konasana)

With your back on the floor and your legs stretched up on the wall, inhale and stretch through your heels.

Exhale and stretch the legs out to the sides, bringing them out and down as far as possible on the wall.

Continue to stretch through your heels, placing your hands on your thighs to keep your legs straight. (See Figure 11.6.)

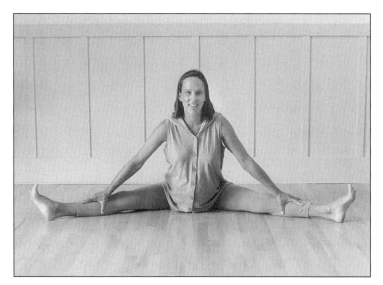

Figure 11.7
If difficult to lie on your back, do Wide-Angled Sitting Pose

Breathe and hold for one minute.

Now relax your arms on the floor out to the sides with your palms facing up.

Breathe and relax your entire pelvic area for up to four minutes.

If you have difficulty lying on your back during the last few months of pregnancy, do Wide-Angled Sitting Pose. (See Figure 11.7 and Figures 8.9 and 8.10, page 119.)

✔ **Elise's Note:** These two poses stretch the groin and inner thigh muscles, which help to ease the delivery of your child. Doing these poses with the legs up the wall gets you off your feet, which is a great relief when carrying all that extra weight!

Sitting Twist (*Bharadvajasana*)

Sit on the floor with your legs straight out in front of you. Bend your left knee and place the top of your left foot to the side of your left buttock, with your toes in a straight line with your calf and heel.

Bend your right knee and slide your right leg under your left thigh toward your lower leg, so that the inner ankle of your left foot fits into the instep of your right foot.

Be sure to keep your hips even, with your left buttock remaining on the floor. If you cannot do this, place a blanket under your right buttock to even your hips.

Inhale and lift up through your spine, aligning your head with your upper body. Exhale and twist to the right, bringing your left hand to your right knee and your right hand to the floor behind your back. (See Figure 11.8.)

Breathe and continue to twist to the right. Be sure your neck and head stay in line with your upper body. Do not lead the twist with your neck and head.

Hold for one minute.

With an exhalation, release your hands and come back to center. Reverse the pose and repeat on the opposite side.

This twist helps to relieve middle and lower back tension that often occurs from the baby pulling the abdomen forward and, as a result, tenses the back muscles.

✔ **Elise's Note:** Hurray! This is one twist you can do when you are pregnant. For all of the others, the baby will get in your way.

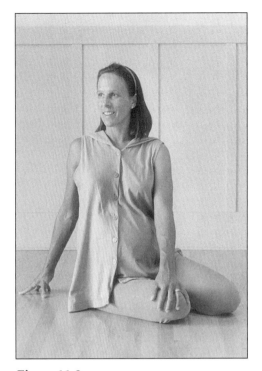

Figure 11.8
Exhale and twist to the right, bringing your left hand to your right knee and your right hand to the floor behind your back

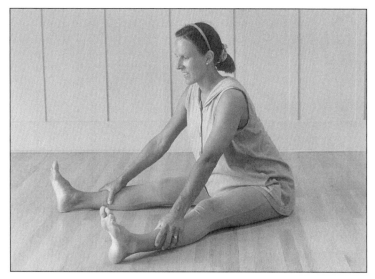

Figure 11.9
Full Forward Bend with the feet placed eighteen inches apart

You can also try Full Forward Bend from the "Menstrual Cycle Relief" section. (See Figure 11.3, page 186.) Make sure to do this pose with your feet placed eighteen inches apart. (See Figure 11.9.) You'll stretch the buttocks, hips, and hamstrings, which need relief from carrying the extra weight.

Healthy Menopause

This next section contains poses to help reduce the physical and mental effects of this "next stage" of life. Please choose the ones you feel are best suited for you. We have listed them in the order we think is the best progression.

Also, the following are some suggested poses that you will find in the other sections of the book. Again, choose the ones you feel are best suited for you.

- Wide-Angle Standing Pose—see Chapter 8, pages 115–116
- Bridging on Wall to Shoulder Stand— see Chapter 10, pages 174–177

- Reclined Bound Angle—see Chapter 12, pages 210–211
- Lazy Shoulder Stand—see Chapter 12, pages 212–213
- Reclined Hero—see pages 181–183
- Head to Knee Pose—see pages 183–185
- Full Forward Bend—see pages 185–186

Elbow Stretch on the Wall

Stand facing the wall, with your feet parallel and hip-width apart. Interlace your fingers, keeping your elbows shoulder-width apart.

Inhale and bring your forearms to the wall, keeping the elbows shoulder-width apart. Be sure to keep the elbows in line with your shoulders and keep your fingers relaxed.

Exhale and walk your feet back, keeping them parallel and hip-width apart. Inhale and bend from your hips, stretching your back and keeping your elbows and forearms on the wall. (See Figure 11.10.)

Exhale and stretch your armpits toward the floor, pushing the shoulder blades toward the front of your body. Keep your head in line with the upper arms.

Continue to stay in the posture for ten breaths, opening the chest and releasing the back.

Slowly exhale, releasing your arms from the wall, coming back to a standing position, and relaxing your arms at your sides.

This stretch opens the chest and gives you a feeling of being more open. As we age, gravity starts to bring us down and sometimes we even feel emotionally depressed. This definitely gives you a lift in life. You can also try Downward Facing Dog. (See Figures 10.1 and 10.2, pages 161–163.)

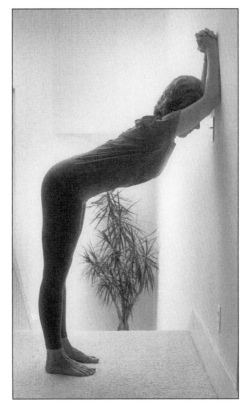

Figure 11.10
Bend from your hips, stretching your back, keeping your elbows and forearms on the wall

Downward Facing Dog
with One Leg Up
(Adho Mukha Svanasana)

Lie on your stomach, with your toes touching a wall. Your palms should be flat on the floor under your shoulders, spreading your fingers out equally. Be sure that your middle fingers are facing directly forward. Your fingertips should be at the edge of your shoulders.

Inhale, exhale, and press down with your palms, lifting your body up so that you are on your hands and knees.

Curl your toes so that you are on the balls of your feet. Bring the lower back into its natural concave curve, with the buttocks bones lifting to the ceiling.

Inhale and exhale, pressing down through the palms and lift from the tailbone, bringing the knees off of the floor, with the heels pressing into the wall. Continue to press down through your palms, particularly through the knuckles at the base of your index and middle fingers.

Stretch up through your arms, spine, and pelvis to your buttocks bones as you stretch back through your legs. Release your neck and head.

Inhale and exhale, lifting your right leg up the wall, placing the ball of the foot on the wall in line with your right hip. (See Figure 11.11, page 195.) Press down with your palms and lift up through your arms, spine, and legs through your heel.

Breathe and hold for thirty seconds, building up to one minute.

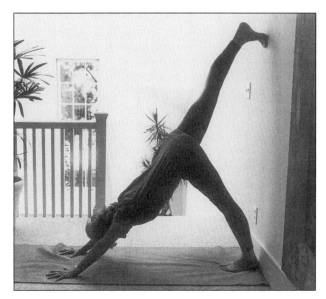

Figure 11.11
Lift your right leg up the wall, placing the ball of the foot on the wall, in line with your right hip

If your shoulders come forward and your back rounds, bend your left knee to bring the chest toward the wall and your spine in its natural concave curve for a deeper stretch of the entire body. As your practice, you will be able to slowly straighten your knee, keeping the alignment of your spine.

Inhale, exhale, and bring the right leg down to the floor. Now bring both knees to the floor and relax in Child's Pose. (See page 53 and Figure 8.14, page 109.)

Repeat on the opposite side.

Variation

If you want a deeper shoulder stretch, interlace your fingers and bring your forearms to the floor, shoulder-width apart.

Come up into Dog Pose with your forearms on the floor, stretching your chest toward your legs. You may lift one leg up the wall. Repeat on the opposite side.

✔ **Elise's Note:** Inversions are very important to do during menopause to help regulate hormones, and this pose is a great preparation for a head stand. You can begin to experience the benefits of inverted poses, which stimulate the pituitary and pineal glands and govern the whole glandular system. It also increases circulation of the blood throughout the body, creating a feeling of vitality. It also stimulates clear thinking.

Child's Pose into a Bolster or Blankets

Get three blankets and fold each into a double fold. (See Figure 12.1, page 200.) Or use a yoga bolster. Place in front of you.

Kneel and sit on your heels, with your knees at the sides of the blankets, bringing your blankets between your thighs.

Inhale and lift up through your spine. Exhale and bend over, lying your right cheek on the blankets. Bring your arms out in front at the sides of the blankets with your palms facing up. (See Figure 11.12, page 197.)

Breathe and relax for two minutes.

Turn your head to the other side and breathe and relax for two minutes.

✔ **Elise's Note:** After the last invigorating pose, this is the perfect position to take. During this stage of our life, it is important to take time to remove stress and relax. This is the ultimate fetal yoga position to do that. Return to the womb.

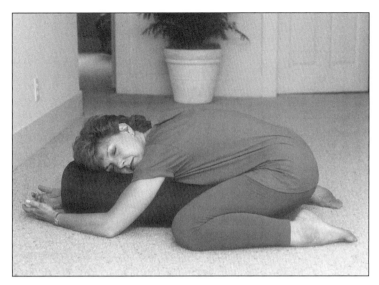

Figure 11.12
With the blankets between your thighs, bend over, laying your right cheek on the blankets and bringing your arms out to the sides

Relaxation *(Savasana)*

Get three blankets and one towel. Fold one blanket into a triple fold. (See Figure 12.1, page 200.) Fold the other two blankets into squares.

Sit down so that the long blanket (triple fold) is behind you, place a blanket square on each side of your thighs, and place a towel where you will place your head.

Bend your knees so that the soles of your feet come together, forming a diamond shape with your legs. Drop your knees so the outer sides of your thighs and calves lie on the folded blanket squares. If you have tight inner thighs and your legs do not touch the blankets, fold the blankets again to make them higher or get additional blankets or pillows.

Lay your spine down lengthwise on top of the long folded blanket, placing the back of your head on the towel so that you can drop your chin toward your chest.

Let your arms drop down at a forty-five degree angle away from your body. Let your shoulders fall away from the blanket and let your legs relax.

You may record this on audio tape.

Lying on your back, focus on relaxing your body into the blankets and floor. Observe your breath flowing deep down into your belly.

On your next exhalation, feel all of the organs in your lower pelvic region relax. Feel your bladder, uterus, and all of your reproductive organs relax.

Slowly breathe in and out and feel yourself sinking deeper and deeper into the floor.

Feel yourself connecting with Mother Earth and all of life around you and let all of the boundaries dissolve.

Invite peace and well-being into your mind and your entire body.

When you are ready, take a deep breath, gently move your fingers and toes, stretch out and open your eyes. Now bring your knees toward your chest, roll over to your side, and using your hands, push back up to a sitting position.

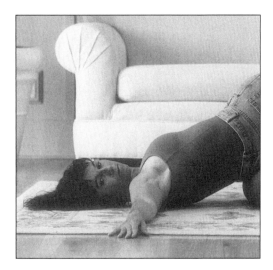

chapter 12

Restore Calm and Relieve Stress

Do you ever feel . . .

. . . someone must have elected you "caretaker" of everyone and everything when you were not in the room? Your "to do" list is endless. You never seem to have time for yourself. You cannot remember the last time you even tried to take a break to relax.

These restorative poses not only relax the body but also calm the nerves and still the mind. By focusing on your breathing in these poses, you can take a break from the thoughts that crowd your day.

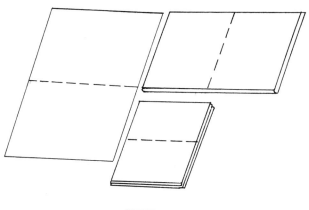

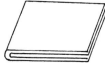

Primary Fold
*Open the blanket and fold
in half three times.
Dimensions: 1″ x 21″ x 28″*

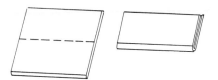

Double Fold
*Start with the primary fold,
then fold in half lengthwise.
Dimensions: 2.5″ x 10″ x 28″*

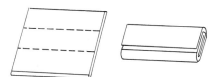

Triple Fold
*Start with the primary fold, then
fold two more times lengthwise.
Dimensions: 5″ x 7.5″ x 28″*

Figure 12.1
Blanket chart illustrating the three
basic folds: primary, double, and triple

When you complete this series, you will have an improved ability to think and remain relaxed and balanced.

You can do these poses at the end of the day or anytime you need a quick break. They can be done as a series of stretches or you can pick the one that feels right for the moment. Remember, if you don't give yourself a break, nobody else will either. So breathe and stretch. You deserve it!

For many of the following poses, you'll need some blankets folded in specific ways. Use the blanket chart shown in Figure 12.1 that illustrates how to do three basic folds: primary, double, and triple. The type of fold or folds required for a pose will be indicated at the beginning of the instructions.

The folds progress from a primary fold to a double or a triple fold. Since most of the poses will require the blanket(s) to be in a double or triple fold, it helps to have each of the blankets folded into a primary fold before beginning this series of stretches.

✔ **Equipment Note:** Two to three blankets (in primary folds), a towel, a book or yoga block, a belt, and a bed. (A yoga bolster is optional.)

Breathing

Now that you have decided to take a relaxation break and restore yourself . . .

Take a blanket and fold it into a triple fold. (See Figure 12.1.) If you are using a thin blanket that does not create a five-inch height, use two blankets. Fold another blanket (or towel) in half and place it at the end of the first.

Sit down so that the first blanket is behind you, with the second blanket at the far end. Lay your spine down lengthwise on top of the first blanket, placing the back of your head on the second blanket so that you can drop you chin slightly toward your chest.

Let your arms drop down at a forty-five degree angle away from your body, palms facing up. Let your shoulders fall away from the blanket and let your legs relax.

As you inhale, fill your belly, ribs, and lungs with air, all the way to your collarbone. Exhale and release your breath from top to bottom, releasing your lungs, ribs, and belly.

Place your hands on your rib cage, with your fingers pointing in toward each other and the heels of your hands on your sides. As the ribs move with your inhalation, see if you can expand your ribs out to the sides, letting the breath expand into your palms and fingers, feeling your breath move from the sides to the front.

Bring your hands back down to your sides and practice feeling an equal balance between your inhalations and exhalations.

You can stay in this pose for five minutes, breathing and relaxing.

If you feel tightness in your lower back, put another blanket or yoga bolster under your knees.

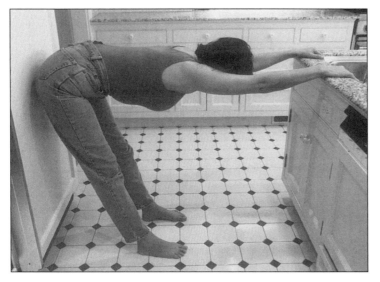

Figure 12.2

Part one: pull backwards, bending at your hips, keeping your neck in line with your spine and chin down

Stretching

Three-Part Pull

Part one: Stand in front of a fence, a railing, or a kitchen sink. Grab onto the kitchen sink (or fence, railing) with both hands shoulder-width apart, and walk the feet back until the spine is parallel to the floor and the feet are directly under the hips.

Walk your feet forward twelve inches in front of your hips and pull backwards away from the sink, bending at your hips. Keep the neck in line with your spine, not allowing your chin to lift up. Feel the entire spine being lengthened by the pull. (See Figure 12.2.)

Breathe and hold for thirty seconds.

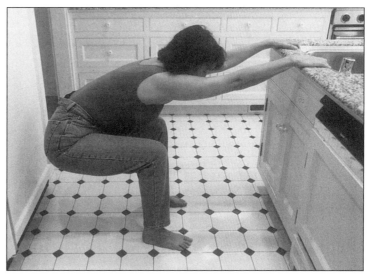

Figure 12.3
Part two: with the heels forward, bend the knees and continue to pull back, stretching your middle back and side ribs

Part two: Bring your heels forward where your toes were, and bend the knees into a right angle, with your thighs parallel to the floor and your knees directly above your heels. Be sure that your front ribs stretch toward the front of your thighs. (See Figure 12.3.)

Continue to pull back, stretching your middle back and side ribs.

Breathe and hold for thirty seconds.

Part three: Walk the feet forward a few more inches, keeping your heels on the floor. Bring your buttocks down toward the floor in a squat. (See Figure 12.4, page 204.)

Pull back again, keeping the buttocks down, and feel the lower back being stretched.

Breathe and hold for thirty seconds.

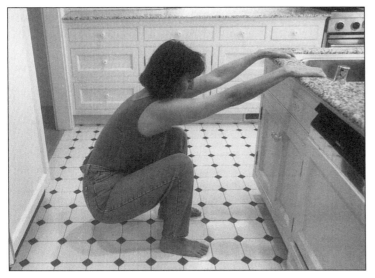

Figure 12.4
Part three: bring the buttocks down in a squat, pulling back again, feeling the lower back being stretched

To come up, inhale and slowly straighten the legs, stretching back through your hips and keeping your arms straight.

✔ **Carol's Note:** This stretch is very easy and you can really feel the stretch in the spine and back muscles.

Lying Over Bolster or Bed

Get two blankets and fold each into a double fold. (See Figure 12.1, page 200.) Or you may use a yoga bolster. Lie down on your back, with your shoulders over the far edge of the blanket or bolster so that your armpits are in line with the edge. Your shoulder blades should be flat on the blankets, with the tops of your shoulders rolling toward the floor.

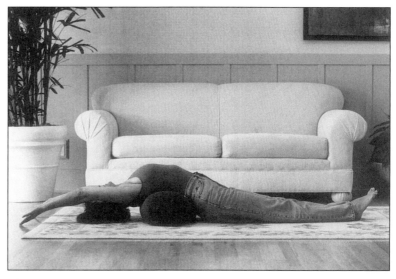

Figure 12.5
Stretch your arms over your head while stretching your pelvis, legs, and heels in the opposite direction

Slowly release your head down to the floor so that the crown of your head touches the floor.

Stretch your arms over your head, extending through your fingers. (See Figure 10.5.) Stretch your pelvis, legs, and heels in the opposite direction and breathe into the mid-chest, expanding the ribs in all directions.

Breathe and relax for two minutes.

Variation

You can also try this pose lying over the edge of your bed in the same position. (See Figure 10.6, page 206.)

This position opens the chest for breathing and encourages better posture since we are often rounding our backs and leaning forward in many daily tasks. It is important each day to go in the

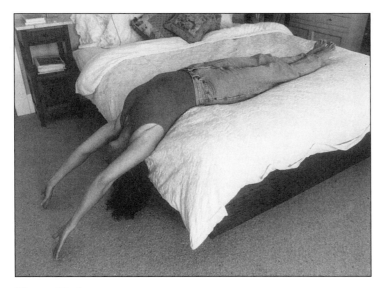

Figure 12.6
Instead of using a bolster, you can do the pose lying on
your bed

opposite direction in order to realign ourselves in a balanced, open posture. Also, this helps with kyphosis, or extreme rounded thoracic (mid-back) spine.

✔ **Elise's Note:** If you're stiff in the neck and the crown of your head does not touch the floor, you may place a second blanket on the floor to support the head. Also, if your shoulders are tight and the hands do not touch the floor, you may bend the elbows and cross the arms at the elbows, lengthening the upper arms and elbows out and down toward the floor.

✔ **Carol's Note:** This is a wonderful way to treat yourself!

Twist on Bolster
(Jatara Parivartanasana)

Get two blankets and fold them into a double fold. (See Figure 12.1, page 200.) You may also use a yoga bolster. Lie down on your back, with your buttocks on the blankets or bolster and your shoulders on the floor. Place your legs hip-width apart, with your knees directly over your heels and your feet parallel. Hold on to the edges of the blanket.

Lift your buttocks slightly from the blanket or bolster, shifting your hips to the right so that your right outer hip lines up with your right shoulder.

Inhale and exhale, lifting the knees toward your chest and aligning your thighs with the blanket. Inhale and stretch your arms out at shoulder height.

Exhale and twist the legs over to the left until you lay your left thigh on the blanket. Keep your head aligned with the middle of your body. Be sure that your lower back is in its natural curve.

Place your left hand on your right thigh to move your right hip so that your right knee lines up with your left knee. Your pelvis should be perpendicular to the floor. Place your right hand on your sacrum (last five fused vertebrae of the spine) to ensure that your pelvis is perpendicular.

Stretch your right arm back out to shoulder height and drop your right shoulder toward the floor.

Gently turn your head to the right and make sure that your right shoulder has dropped to the floor. (See Figure 12.7, page 208.)

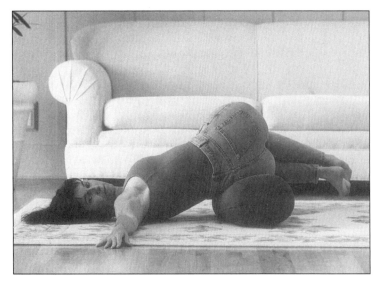

Figure 12.7
With your knees aligned to the left and your pelvis perpendicular to the floor, drop your right shoulder to the floor, gently turning your head to the right

Breathe and hold for two minutes.

Inhale and exhale, lifting your legs back to center. Place your feet on the floor to shift your hips to the left side, twisting to the right.

Repeat the entire sequence.

When finished, bring your left hand over to the right side and press your palms down to bring your upper body to an upright position.

Variation

As you become more comfortable with this pose, you may straighten your legs by stretching out through your heels, keeping your feet together. Your legs will be at a right angle to your upper body.

This is a relaxing yet beneficial twist to help relieve lower back tension.

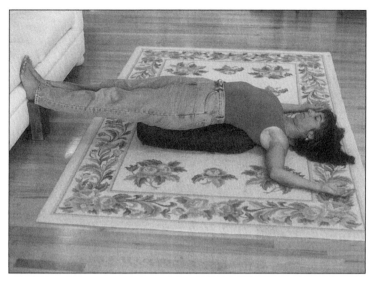

Figure 12.8
Pressing your feet into the wall or sofa, bend your elbows at a right angle with palms facing up

Bridge on Bolster Supported (Setu Bandha Sarvangasana)

Get two blankets and fold each into a double fold. (See Figure 12.1, page 200.) Or you may use a yoga bolster. Also get a hardcover book or a yoga block and place it upright against a wall or an upholstered chair or sofa. Place the blanket lengthwise, twelve or more inches away from the book.

Lie on your back on the blanket, with the tip or base of your shoulder blades on the edge of the blanket. The tops of your shoulders should rest on the floor.

Place your feet on the wall or sofa so that your heels rest on the top of the book or yoga block. Press into the wall or sofa.

Place your arms at shoulder height and bend your elbows at a right angle, with your palms facing the ceiling. (See Figure 12.8.)

Breathe and hold for five minutes.

Slowly bend the knees and bring the feet to the floor. Roll to your right side and use your hands to bring your upper body to an upright position.

This is the most relaxing pose for the nervous system, with the body supine yet the chest open. It also helps improve your posture and decreases rounded shoulders and kyphosis.

✔ **Elise's Note:** If you feel discomfort in your lower back, raise your legs higher on the wall or onto the seat of the sofa. Also, placing a belt tightly around your upper thighs will decrease any discomfort. As you practice this regularly, your back will bend backwards more easily and the discomfort will disappear.

Reclined Bound Angle Pose (Supta Baddha Konasana)

Get two blankets and fold each into a double fold. (See Figure 12.1, page 200.) Or you may use a yoga bolster. Place the blankets or the bolster lengthwise.

Sit on the floor, with your back on the edge of the blankets. Lie down on the blankets lengthwise, with a towel to support your head. Let your arms relax down by your sides, palms facing up.

Bend your knees and bring the bottoms of your feet together. Let your knees drop to the sides, away from your body. (See Figure 12.9, page 211.)

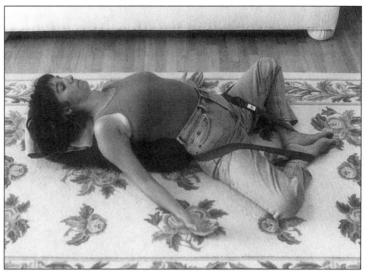

Figure 12.9
Bringing the bottoms of your feet together, let your knees drop to the sides . . . to increase the stretch, you may use a belt around your feet and back

Press through the heels, stretching the knees away from each other and pressing toward the floor.

Breathe and hold for five minutes.

You may use your hands to help slowly bring your knees back together. Roll to your right side and use your hands to bring your upper body to an upright position. If your inner thighs are tight and your knees are far off the floor, you may place blankets or pillows under your legs for support.

Variation

If you want to increase the stretch in the inner thighs, you may place a belt around your feet and back as shown in Figure 12.9.

This pose opens the chest and diaphragm as well as stretches the inner thighs.

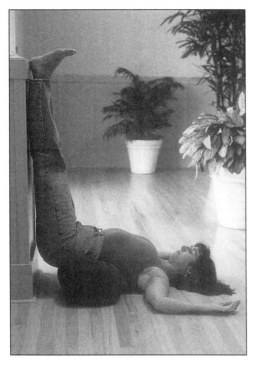

Figure 12.10
With your shoulders on the floor and buttocks dropped slightly, bend the elbows to form right angles

Lazy Shoulder Stand (Viparita Karani)

Get two blankets and fold each into a double fold. (See Figure 12.1, page 200.) Or you may use a yoga bolster. Place the blankets six inches away from a wall.

To get into position, lie sideways with both buttocks bones touching the wall. Swing your legs up the wall, bringing your lower back onto the blankets or bolster, dropping the buttocks slightly to the floor. Your shoulders should touch the floor, with your lower ribs on the edge of the blankets or bolster. The buttocks drop slightly toward the floor, creating a softness in your groin and belly.

Bend the elbows, placing the upper arms in line with your shoulders and your forearms at a right angle. With your palms facing up to the ceiling, relax your fingers. (See Figure 12.10.)

Close your eyes, imagining that you are dropping your vision down toward your cheekbones.

Breathe and rest in this pose for up to five minutes.

Bend your legs and place your hands on your shins, bringing your knees toward your chest. Exhale, stretching your lower back. Roll gently from side to side, massaging your lower back.

Roll to the right side, using your hands to bring the upper body to an upright position.

This position also opens the chest and decreases rounded shoulders. In addition, it has similar benefits as the shoulder stand, balancing the glandular system and calming the mind, but can be done with less effort.

✔ **Elise's Note:** If you feel any discomfort in the lower back, place only one blanket underneath you or just lie with your buttocks flat on the floor.

✔ **Carol's Note:** This is the pose to do if you've been on your feet all day and need to revitalize before a night on the town!

Twist Facing Bolster (Supta Bharadvajasana)

Get two blankets and fold them into a double fold. (See Figure 12.1, page 200.) Or you may use a yoga bolster.

Sit on the floor, with your legs straight out in front of you and the short edge of your blanket next to your right hip (perpendicular to your legs).

Bend your left knee and place the top of your left foot to the side of your left buttock, with your toes in a straight line with your calf and heel.

Bend your right knee and slide your right leg under your left thigh toward your lower leg so that the inner ankle of your left foot fits into the instep of your right foot. Be sure to keep your right hip aligned with the edge of the blanket.

Before lying over the bolster or blankets, it is important to do this twist from a seated position. (See Figure 11.8, page 191.)

Inhale and lift up through your spine, aligning your head with your upper body. Exhale and twist to the right, bringing your left hand to your right knee and your right hand behind your right buttock.

Breathe and continue to twist to the right. Be sure your neck and head stay in line with your upper body. Do not lead the twist with your neck and head. Hold for five breaths.

Bring your left hand to the left side of your blanket and your right hand to the right side. Shift onto the right side of your right hip. Bring your left shoulder forward so that the chest directly faces your blanket.

Inhale and exhale, pressing the right palm to the floor as you continue to twist the left side of the upper body forward, and lower your chest to the blanket, placing your left cheekbone on your blanket. (See Figure 12.11, page 215.) Let your arms relax at shoulder height, with your elbows bent and your palms facing the ceiling.

Breathe and relax for five minutes.

Place your palms on the floor, pressing down to lift your upper body off of the blanket.

Repeat the sequence to twist to the left side.

This is a wonderful twist of the spine and relieves lower back tightness. It also frees the ribs and mid-back to breathe deeper and with more ease.

✔ **Elise's Note:** If your head does not comfortably turn away from your legs, you may add a small blanket or pillow to add more height or you may lay your cheekbone down with your head facing the same direction as your legs.

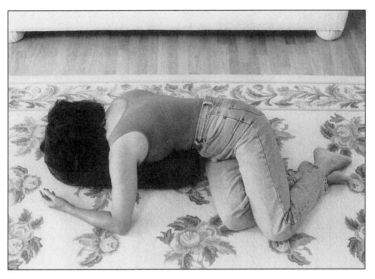

Figure 12.11
Continue to twist the left side of the upper body forward and lower your chest to the blanket, placing your left cheekbone to your blanket

Relaxation *(Savasana)*

Get a towel and two blankets. Fold each of the two blankets into a triple fold. (See Figure 12.1, page 200.) Fold the towel in half.

Sit down so that one blanket is behind you and place the towel across the far end of the blanket. Place the second blanket under your knees.

Lie down lengthwise along the blanket folded behind you and support your head with the towel. Let your arms drop down at a forty-five degree angle away from your body. Let your shoulders fall away from the blanket and let your legs relax.

Now record this on audio tape.

Begin to feel your entire body relaxing from your head all the way down to the tips of your toes.

As you inhale, feel your breath flowing into every pore, every cell of your entire body. Exhale and feel the deep release from every cell and every pore of your entire body.

As you inhale, feel the restoring energy flowing into every part of your body. Exhale and feel all of your exhaustion, all of your stress, all of your tension dissolve away. Feel your nerve impulses slowing down.

Listen to the steady rhythm of your heartbeat throughout your body. Listen to your heart slow down and relax. Feel your brain letting go of all stressful thoughts and invite peace and well-being into your mind and your entire body.

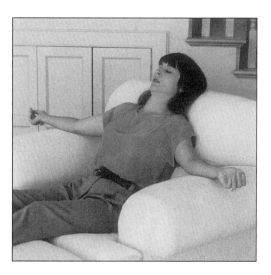

chapter   1 3

Relax and Find Balance in Your Life

Do you ever feel . . .

. . . you would love to have a few minutes each day to spend relaxing? You would love to, but you feel guilty just doing nothing. How can you justify wasting time relaxing?

Studies have shown that relaxing five or ten minutes a day will lower your blood pressure, making you healthier. Even if you do not take time to do your twenty minutes of stretching, you can benefit from taking a few minutes to relax each day. Your health is more important than all the things you have to do. Similar studies have proven that relaxation actually helps you focus on the tasks you want to complete. In other words, by relaxing you become more productive.

We have created three visualizations: stress reduction, achieving success, and health and vitality. Each of these visualizations start with relaxing the body. Then we give you some words to create positive images in your mind. Finally, we give you words for "coming back," which means gently returning to full consciousness.

We suggested in each of the preceding chapters that you record the relaxation session instructions on a tape recorder to lead you through the process anytime, anywhere. You can do the same thing with these visualizations. (When recording, you may choose to put the visualizations into the first person.) It is important to give yourself enough time for each component. Don't rush. You can even leave some quiet time between the instructions for the different components.

Remember, you are worth it. You may do these sessions anytime you feel you need it or at the end of your yoga stretches. Enjoy!

✔ **Equipment Note:** You might need a yoga bolster or two blankets and a tape recorder.

Preparation

You may do these relaxation sessions sitting in a comfortable chair or lying down.

Sitting

If you are sitting in an office or dining room chair, let your back rest against the back of the chair so that you feel no tension. Have your feet parallel to each other and flat on the floor, hip-width apart.

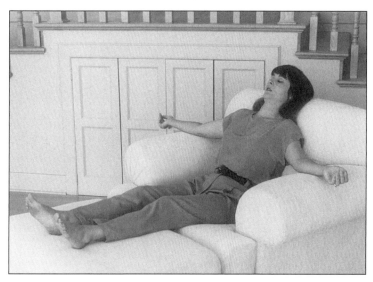

Figure 13.1
If your chair has an armrest, place your forearms on the armrest with the palms of your hands facing up

If you have a chair with an ottoman or comfortable leg rest, let your legs relax straight out in front of you. (See Figure 13.1.)

If your chair does not have an armrest, place your hands on your thighs, with your palms facing up.

If your chair does have an armrest, place your forearms on the armrest, with the palms facing up. (See Figure 13.1.) Keep your head centered so it is not leaning in one direction or the other.

Lying Down

Make sure that your body is aligned by imagining a string running straight through the middle of your body and out the top of your head.

Bring your arms down by your sides, approximately twelve inches away from your thighs, with the palms facing up.

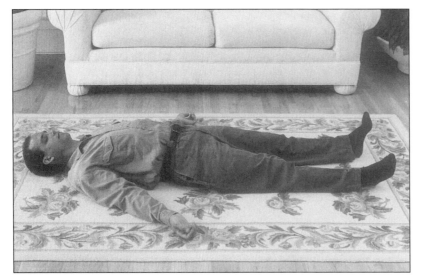

Figure 13.2
Make sure that your body is aligned by imagining a string running straight through the middle of your body and out the top of your head

To properly place your feet, begin by bending your knees and placing your feet flat on the floor in order to relax your lower back.

Slowly inhale and slide your right heel out, straightening your leg and stretching through your right heel. Now exhale and let your entire leg relax, letting your foot fall naturally to the right side.

Repeat on the left side by stretching out through your left heel and letting your left foot fall naturally to the left side.

Now raise your head up slightly to check the alignment of your body. Be sure that the "string" running through the middle of your body is straight. (See Figure 13.2.)

Now hold the back of your head in your hands and stretch the back of your neck, placing your head on the floor, making sure your head is centered. This is just like the feeling you created at the beginning of your stretching practice with Palm Tree Pose in Chapter 2. (See pages 18–19.)

! **Caution:** If you feel any tension in your lower back, bend your knees and place a yoga bolster or two blankets under your knees for support. Then do the relaxation and visualization sessions with your knees bent over the bolster or blankets to protect your lower back.

Relaxation Visualizations

Stress Reduction

You may feel stress creep up and take over during a busy day. You may want to do something good for yourself like the stretches in this book. However, you may find it difficult to stop what you are doing and take a break. To stop the stress, break the pattern of anxiety and change your state of mind. You may choose to do this visualization before beginning your stretching routine. Of course, you can do this visualization anytime before, after, or separate from any stretches to completely relax.

Relaxing

Sit or lie down in a comfortable position. Close your eyes and begin to relax every muscle in your body, from the tips of your toes to the crown of your head. Feel your body relaxing now as you begin to sink deeper and deeper into relaxation. Relax and let go of all thoughts and all emotions. Just feel your thoughts dissolving now as you continue to relax even deeper and deeper.

Relax your body now, beginning with the soles of your feet. Relax your heels, your toes, your shins, and your calves. Now feel that soothing relaxation begin to move up into your knees, your thighs, and your lower pelvic region. Feel all of your buttock muscles relaxing as you continue to drop deeper and deeper into total relaxation.

Relax your reproductive organs, your bladder, your intestines, your kidneys, your liver, and your stomach. Now feel the soothing relaxation begin to move up into your chest, relaxing your lungs, ribs, and heart.

Observe your breathing flowing gently in and out, bringing energy and relaxation to your entire body.

Feel your lower back, your mid-back, and your upper back muscles and spine soften and relax deeper and deeper. Feel the soothing relaxation move up your spine and into your neck and shoulder muscles. Feel all of the neck and shoulder muscles relax, feeling all of your responsibilities dissolving away. Feel the relaxation move down your arms and all of the way out to your fingertips. Observe your breathing flowing in and out, in and out, bringing energy and relaxation to your entire body.

Now feel the soothing relaxation move into your facial muscles, relaxing your chin, jaw, tongue, even your teeth and gums. Let the relaxation move into your nose, ears, and eyes. Allow your eyes to drop deeply into your eye sockets, allowing your vision to drop downward to your cheekbones. Feel your forehead muscles relaxing now as you feel your brain drop from your forehead to the back of your skull, releasing all of your thoughts.

Feel the soothing relaxation move all the way up through the crown of your head. Observe your breathing flowing in and out, in and out, completely relaxing your entire body.

Visualization

Now that you are completely relaxed, visualize yourself in a situation where you feel unwanted pressure. As you see this pressure beginning to surround you, see yourself being protected by a magic shield. This shield will protect you from all unwanted pressures, all of your stressful thoughts, all of your "to do" lists, all of your feelings of anxiety about what is happening around you. See yourself protected so that none of the pressure can invade you. See the pressure bounce off and away. See all of the pressure just bounce off and away.

You are relaxed and comfortable and have all of the time you need to take care of each situation. The pressure that is coming at you just bounces off and away. Now you see yourself calm and relaxed. You know that you can do what will make you feel healthy and more relaxed. You know exactly what to do, and you have the time to do it.

Visualize yourself beginning to do a stretching routine that will make you feel even more healthy and more relaxed. See yourself doing the stretches, getting more open, more relaxed, and gaining more energy as you go through your routine. Now you can see yourself completing the routine, feeling that you have restored your health, relaxed your body, and calmed your mind. You feel so pleased with yourself, so happy with yourself, that you are doing what you need to do for yourself.

Now visualize yourself protected and able to handle any pressures, any thoughts, any feelings that may come your way. You now know that you can cope with each situation in turn, and you have the time you need to focus on whatever you choose to accomplish. You can handle any situation with a calm attitude. Relax for just another moment, seeing yourself calm and capable and ready to begin to return to this space and time.

Coming Back

Relax for just another moment now. Observe your breathing. Breathe in and out, feeling your body begin to move now, expanding your chest, ribs, and lungs. Exhale and feel a deep release of all of the air, dropping back down to the floor. Now begin to slowly move your fingers and wiggle your toes. Begin to stretch out and become aware of your surroundings. Gently open your eyes and return, feeling completely refreshed and alert.

Achieving Success

To achieve success in anything, you need to have a positive self-image and believe in your ability to accomplish your goals. Use this visualization to challenge your fears of failure and to increase your self-confidence. It is time to encourage yourself to use your talents to the best of your abilities. This visualization works well for anyone wanting to boost their self-esteem regarding business, personal relationships, athletics, or creativity.

Relaxing

Sit or lie down in a comfortable position. Close your eyes and begin to relax every muscle in your body, from the tips of your toes to the crown of your head. Feel your body relaxing as you begin to sink deeper and deeper into relaxation. Relax and let go of all thoughts and all emotions. Just feel your thoughts dissolving as you continue to relax even deeper and deeper.

Relax your body beginning with the soles of your feet. Relax your heels, your toes, your shins, and your calves. Feel that soothing relaxation begin to move up into your knees, thighs, and lower pelvic region. Feel all of your buttock muscles relaxing as you continue to drop deeper and deeper into total relaxation.

Relax your reproductive organs, bladder, intestines, kidneys, liver, and stomach. Feel the soothing relaxation begin to move up into your chest, relaxing your lungs, ribs, and heart. Observe your breathing flowing gently in and out, bringing energy and relaxation to your entire body.

Feel your lower back, your mid-back, and upper back muscles and spine soften and relax deeper and deeper. Feel the soothing relaxation move up your spine and into your neck and shoulder muscles. Feel all of the neck and shoulder muscles relax, feeling all of your responsibilities dissolving away. Feel the relaxation move down your arms, all the way to your fingertips. Observe your breathing flowing in and out, in and out, bringing energy and relaxation to your entire body.

Now feel the soothing relaxation move into your facial muscles, relaxing your chin, jaw, tongue, even your teeth and gums. Let the relaxation move into your nose, ears, and eyes. Allow your eyes to drop deeply into your eye sockets, allowing your vision to drop downward to the cheekbones. Feel your forehead muscles relaxing now, all of your forehead muscles relaxing as you feel your brain drop from your forehead to the back of your skull, releasing all of your thoughts. Feel the soothing relaxation move all the way up through the crown of your head. Observe your breathing flowing in and out, in and out, completely relaxing your entire body.

Visualization

Now that you are completely relaxed, see yourself walking into a private room, your very special room, with a large screen and a computer keyboard. You are going to have the ability to create and record any situation with words and pictures that will appear on your screen. Sit down in your very comfortable chair and feel completely relaxed as you begin to use your special screen to create the positive images of who you are and what you want to accomplish.

Now, begin to see an image of yourself on the screen surrounded by words that describe you. Look at the words. If you want to change any of these descriptions, use the delete button on your keyboard and replace the negative description with one you want to present. You have the ability to change any negative descriptions of yourself to positive ones. As a result of changing the words, see yourself change into a more positive image. Since you have the ability to control the images on the screen, now you can play a video of yourself accomplishing your goals in business, athletics, or a creative task.

At first, you may see yourself concerned with fears, criticism, and an inability to accomplish what you would like to do. Use your control to change the images you see of yourself into someone who is proud of who you are and what you are doing. Imagine yourself happy with the way you look and act. Feel a new sense of self-confidence as you use a new and healthy energy to feel sure of your abilities. You are capable, talented, creative, and have a positive image of yourself. Take a few moments to watch the video and enjoy seeing yourself accomplishing your goals in business, personal relationships, athletics, or creativity. You feel happy and confident and so pleased with yourself. Take a few moments to relax with your images in silence. Relax for just another moment, seeing yourself calm and capable and ready to begin to return to this space and time.

Coming Back

Relax for just another moment now. Observe your breathing. Breathe in and out, feeling your body begin to move now, expanding your chest, ribs, and lungs. Exhale and feel a deep release of all of the air, dropping back down to the floor. Now begin to slowly move your fingers and wiggle your toes. Begin to stretch out and become aware of your surroundings. Gently open your eyes and return feeling completely refreshed and alert.

Health and Vitality

We believe that everyone has the ability to positively affect their own health and well-being. This visualization allows you to create a scene where you take control of your health and make specific improvements. You can increase your energy and vitality by utilizing your own healing powers. Studies have proven that an individual can control pain, counteract illness, and boost the immune system by positive imaging and mental focus.

Relaxing

Sit or lie down in a comfortable position. Close your eyes and begin to relax every muscle in your body, from the tips of your toes to the crown of your head. Feel your body relaxing now as you begin to sink deeper and deeper into relaxation. Relax and let go of all thoughts and all emotions. Just feel your thoughts dissolving as you continue to relax even deeper and deeper.

Relax your body now, beginning with the soles of your feet. Relax your heels, your toes, your shins, and your calves. Feel that soothing relaxation begin to move up into your knees, thighs, and lower pelvic region. Feel all of your buttock muscles relaxing as your continue to drop deeper and deeper into total relaxation.

Relax your reproductive organs, bladder, intestines, kidneys, liver, and stomach. Feel the soothing relaxation begin to move up into your chest, relaxing your lungs, ribs, and heart. Observe your breathing flowing gently in and out, bringing energy and relaxation to your entire body.

Feel your lower back, mid-back, and upper back muscles and spine soften and relax deeper and deeper. Feel the soothing relaxation move up your spine and into your neck and shoulder muscles. Feel all of the neck and shoulder muscles relax, feeling all of your responsibilities dissolving away. Feel the relaxation move down your arms and all the way out to your fingertips.

Observe your breathing flowing in and out, in and out, bringing energy and relaxation to your entire body.

Now feel the soothing relaxation move into your facial muscles, relaxing your chin, jaw, tongue, even your teeth and gums. Let the relaxation move into your nose, ears, and eyes. Allow your eyes to drop deeply into your eye sockets, allowing your vision to drop downward to the cheekbones.

Feel your forehead muscles relaxing now, all of your forehead muscles relaxing as you feel your brain drop from your forehead to the back of your skull, releasing all of your thoughts. Feel the soothing relaxation move all the way up through the crown of your head. Observe your breathing flowing in and out, in and out, completely relaxing your entire body.

Visualization

Now that you are completely relaxed, imagine yourself on a path that will lead you to your very special place. This place can be a soothing place where you feel comfortable, relaxed, and totally serene. You may want to take yourself on a walk in the woods, or to a special beach, or to the mountains, or even to a meadow full of wildflowers. Wherever you choose, this place is a special place to heal and revitalize. Now that you are in your special place, relax and choose a place to sit or lie down where you feel totally relaxed and supported in your surroundings.

Now that you are relaxing in your special place, begin to imagine your healing force taking shape. Your powers could take the shape of a human helper, or an animal friend, or a part of the nature surrounding you that has come to support and heal you. Ask your healing image to help you focus on some part of you that needs to be healed. Ask for help and receive the loving support and healing energy from your special image.

As you inhale, let the healing energy flow in through every pore and every cell of your body. As you exhale, feel the healing energy cleansing and releasing you of all of your "dis-ease." Feel your body restored to good health and feel the increase in positive energy and vitality. You are strong and healthy and fully alive.

Thank your healing image for being there to support and revitalize you. Ask your image to return the next time you need help. Know that your special image will be waiting in your special place every time you need it. Relax for just another moment, seeing yourself calm and capable and ready to begin to return to this space and time.

Coming Back

Relax for just another moment now. Observe your breathing. Breathe in and out, feeling your body begin to move now, expanding your chest, ribs, and lungs. Exhale and feel a deep release of all of the air, dropping back down into the support of the floor. Now begin to slowly move your fingers and wiggle your toes. Begin to stretch out and become aware of your surroundings. Gently open your eyes and return, feeling completely refreshed and alert.

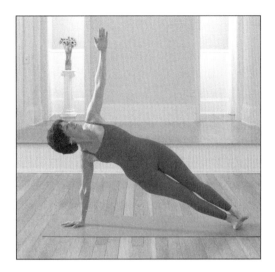

chapter 14

Create Your Own Yoga Practice

Do you ever feel . . .

. . . you should practice yoga but are not sure what poses to choose? Or you want to relieve tension but are not sure what poses would work best? Or you want a well-rounded practice but do not know how to put together the best routine?

Here are eight routines that will help you create your practice from the poses you have learned throughout the book. Choose a fifteen minute routine to energize and center you. Or select a routine to work on a particular area of your body. By following the series of routines throughout the week, you will work all areas of your body. The last routine is designed as a well-rounded practice.

Fifteen Minute Sequence

Focus: These poses comprise a well-rounded sequence that can be done in fifteen minutes. A short practice can be enough of a commitment to make a difference. These poses energize you along with keeping you centered and relaxed throughout the day.

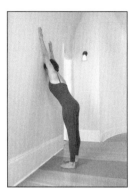

1. Wall Stretch
pages 41–42

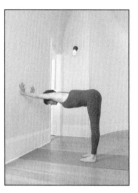

2. Right-Angled Wall Stretch
(Ardha Uttanasana)
pages 108–109

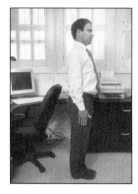

3. Palm Tree Pose
(Tadasana)
page 18

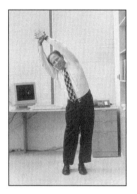

4. Side Stretch with the Wrist
page 23

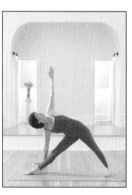

5. Triangle Pose
(Trikonasana)
pages 76–77

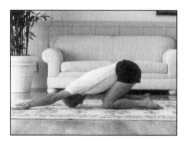

6. Extended Puppy Pose
(Vajrasana)
page 57–58

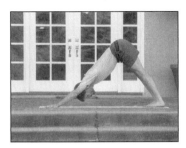 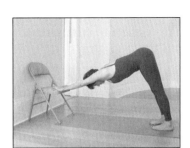 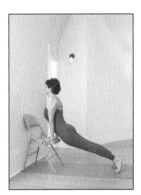

7. Downward Facing Dog
(Adho Mukha Svanasana)
pages 161–163

**8. Downward Facing Dog
with chair**
(Adho Mukha Svanasana)
pages 161–162

**9. Upward Facing Dog
with chair**
*(Urdhva Mukha
Svanasana)*
pages 164–166

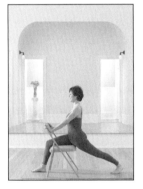 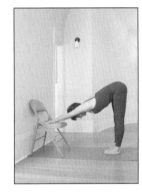

**10. Warrior I
with chair**
(Virabhadrasana I)
pages 138–140

**11. Standing Forward
Bend
with chair**
(Uttanasana)
page 150

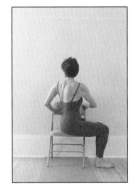 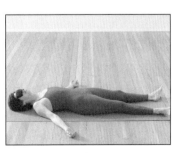

12. Chair Twist
(Chair Bharadvajasana)
page 155

13. Relaxation
(Savasana)
pages 157–158

Monday
Standing Poses: Focus on Legs and Hips

Focus: These poses focus on lengthening and strengthening the legs, energizing the hips and bringing vitality to the spine and entire body. This practice teaches us to stand on our own two feet.

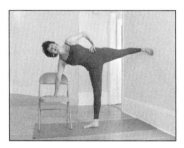 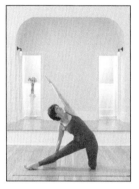 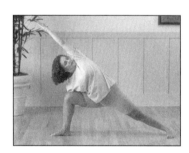

1. Downward Facing Dog
(Adho Mukha Svanasana)
pages 161–163

2. Gate Pose
(Parighasana)
pages 132–133

3. Triangle Pose
(Trikonasana)
pages 76–77

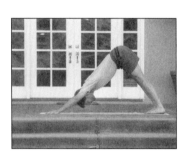 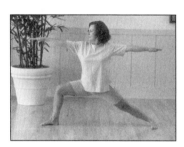 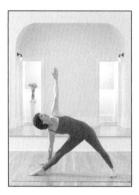

4. Half Moon with chair
(Ardha Chandrasana)
pages 134–135

5. Warrior II
(Virabhadrasana II)
pages 77–78

6. Right-Angled Side Stretch
(Utthita Parsvakonasana)
page 79–81

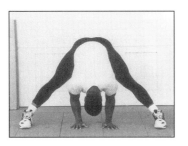

7. Wide-Angled Standing Pose
(Prasarita Padottanasana)
pages 115–117

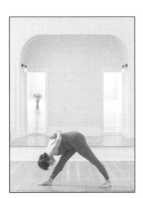

8. One-Legged Hamstring Stretch
(Parsvottanasana)
pages 141–144

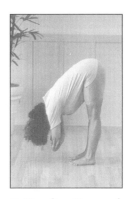

9. Standing Forward Bend
(Uttanasana)
pages 81–82

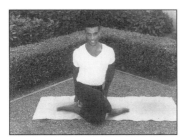

10. Sitting Hip Opener
(Gomukhasana)
pages 122–123

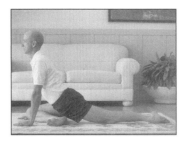

11. Hip Opener
page 235

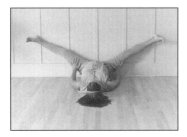

12. Wide-Angled Pose on the wall
(Upavistha Konasana)
pages 189–190

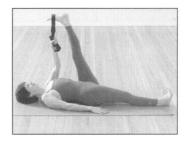

13a. Hamstring Stretch
(Supta Padangustasana)
pages 126–128

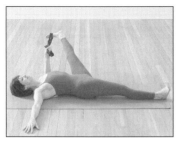

13b. Hamstring Stretch
(Supta Padangustasana)
pages 126–128

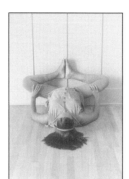

**14. Bound Angle Pose
with legs up wall**
(Baddha Konasana)
pages 187–188

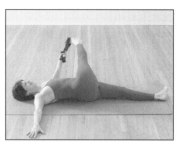

**15. Spinal Twist
and Hip Opener**
*(One-legged Jathara
Parivartanasana)*
pages 156–157

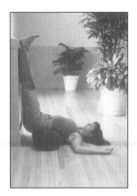

**16. Lazy Shoulder
Stand**
(Viparita Karani)
pages 212–213

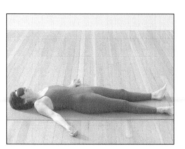

17. Relaxation
(Savasana)
pages 157–158

Tuesday
Lower Back Focus

Focus: These poses focus on relieving tension in the lower back and give you tools to prevent future lower back problems. Maintain the normal curves of the spine as much as possible. The goal is to create flexibility in the hamstrings and hip flexors and strengthen the abdominals and back muscles.

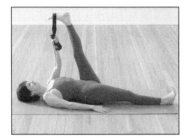

1a. Hamstring Stretch
(Supta Padangusthasana)
pages 126–128

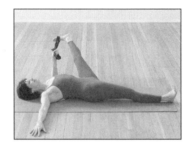

1b. Hamstring Stretch
(Supta Padangusthasana)
pages 126–128

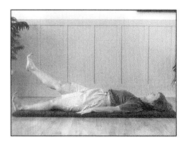

2. Leg Lifts
(Urdhva Prasarita Padasana)
pages 94–95

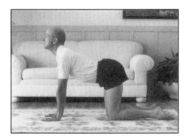

3a. Cat Cow Pelvic Tilts
pages 52–53

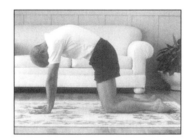

3b. Cat Cow Pelvic Tilts
pages 52–53

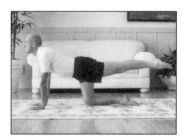

4a. Cat Cow with Leg Extension
pages 54–55

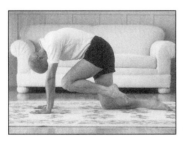

4a. Cat Cow with Leg Extension
pages 54–55

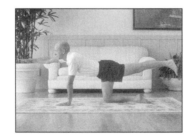

5. Four Point Stabilization
pages 56–57

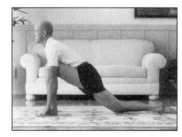

6. Kneeling Lunge
pages 58–59

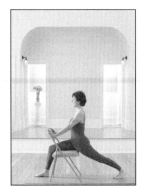

7. Extended Puppy Pose
(Vajrasana)
pages 57– 58

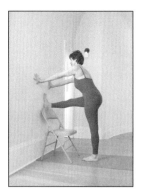

**8a. Standing
Hamstring Stretch &
Inner Thigh Stretch**
*(Utthita Hasta
Padangusthasana I & II)*
pages 114–115

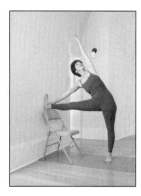

**8b. Standing
Hamstring Stretch &
Inner Thigh Stretch**
*(Utthita Hasta
Padangusthasana I & II)*
pages 148–149

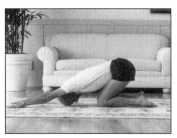

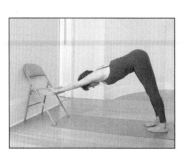

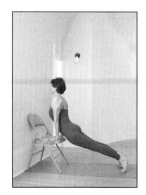

**9. Warrior I
with chair**
(Virabhadrasana I)
pages 138–140

**10. Downward Facing Dog
with chair**
(Adho Mukha Svanasana)
pages 161–162

**11. Upward Facing
Dog
with chair**
*(Urdhva Mukha
Svanasana)*
pages 164–165

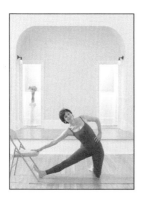

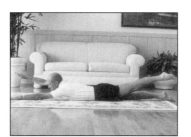

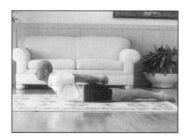

12. Gate Pose
(Parighasana)
pages 132–133

13. Back Strengthener
Variation 1
pages 64–65

14. Back Strengthener
Variation 2
pages 66–67

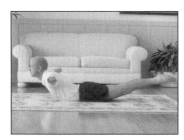

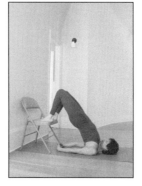

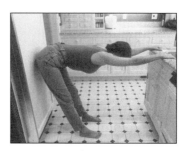

15. Back Strengthener
Variation 3
pages 67–68

16. Bridge Pose
with chair
(Setu Bandha
Sarvangasana)
pages 84–86

17a. Three-Part Pull
pages 202–204

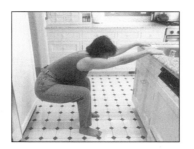

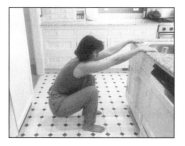

17b. Three-Part Pull
pages 202–204

17c. Three-Part Pull
pages 202–204

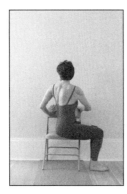

18. Chair Twist
(Chair Bharadvajasana)
page 155

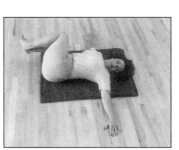

19. Floor Twist
(Jathara Parivartanasana)
pages 83–84

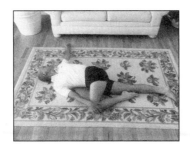

20. Crocodile Twist
pages 68–69

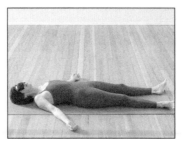

21. Relaxation
(Savasana)
pages 157–158

Wednesday
Shoulders, Neck, and Upper Back Focus

Focus: These poses focus on relieving tension in the neck, shoulders and upper back by creating more flexibility of the back and neck muscles. You also develop strength in the arms to ultimately save the back. Time to let go of all the responsibility that we hold in our shoulders and upper body!

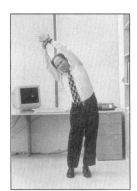

1. Side Stretch with the Wrist
pages 23–24

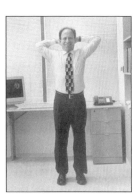

2a. Chest and Neck Stretch
page 24

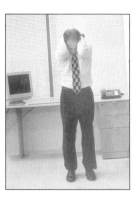

2b. Chest and Neck Stretch
page 24

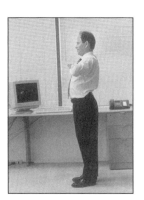

3a. Mid Back Stretch
pages 26–27

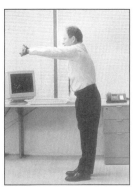

3b. Mid Back Stretch
pages 26–27

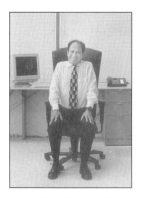

4. Shoulder Rolls
pages 28–29

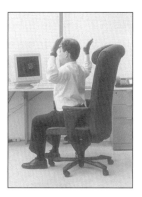

**5. Upper Body
Alignment**
pages 29–30

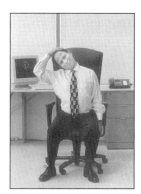

6. Neck Stretch
pages 30–31

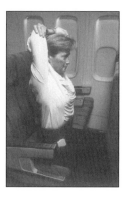

**7. Elbow to Ceiling
Stretch**
pages 37–38

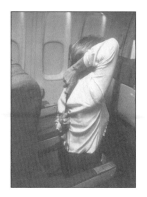

8. Shoulder Stretch
(Gomukhasana)
page 38

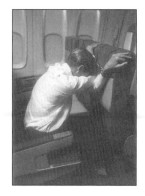

**9. Shoulder Blade
Stretch**
(Garudhasana)
pages 39–40

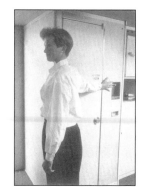

10. Shoulder Twist
pages 43–44

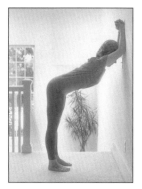

**11. Elbow Stretch
on the Wall**
page 193

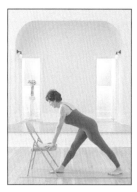

**12. One-Legged
Hamstring Stretch
with chair**
(Parsvottanasana)
pages 141–143

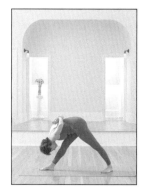

**13. One-Legged
Hamstring Stretch
Classic Pose**
(Parsvottanasana)
pages 142–144

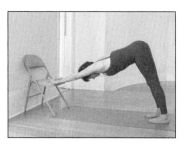

**14. Downward Facing Dog
with chair**
(Adho Mukha Svanasana)
pages 161–162

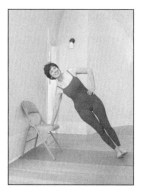

**15. Arm Balance and
Back Strengthener
with chair**
(Vasisthasana)
pages 151–152

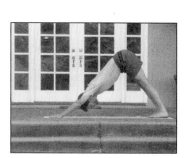

16. Downward Facing Dog
(Adho Mukha Svanasana)
pages 161–163

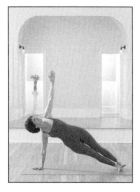

**17. Arm Balance and
Back Strengthener**
(Vasisthasana)
pages 152–153

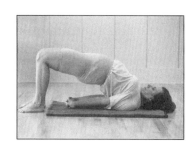

18. Bridge Pose
(Setu Bandha Sarvangasana)
pages 84–86

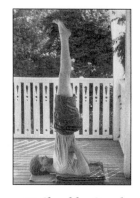

19. Shoulder Stand
*(Salamba
Sarvangasana)*
pages 174–176

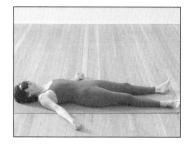

20. Relaxation
(Savasana)
pages 157–158

Thursday
Energize and Open the Heart with Backbends

Focus: These poses focus on creating more flexibility in the mid-back to open and free the heart with the practice of backbends. You also allow more oxygen to enter the lungs, creating a feeling of openness and flexibility to bend in all directions throughout life.

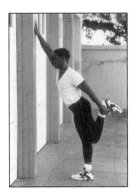

1. Shooting Bow Pose
(Natarajasana)
page 113

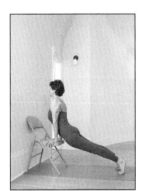

**2. Lying over Bolster
or Bed**
pages 204–206

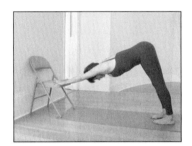

**3. Downward Facing Dog
with chair**
(Adho Mukha Svanasana)
pages 161–162

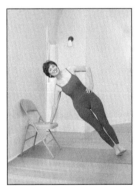

**4. Arm Balance and
Back Strengthener
with chair**
(Vasistasana)
pages 151–152

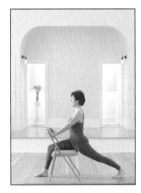

**5. Warrior I
with chair**
(Virabhadrasana)
pages 138–140

**6. Upward Facing Dog
with chair**
*(Urdhva Mukha
Svanasana)*
pages 164–165

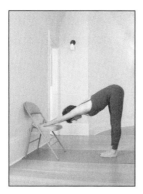

**7. Standing Forward
Bend
with chair**
(Uttanasana)
page 150

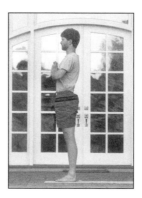

8a. Sun Salutations
pages 167–173

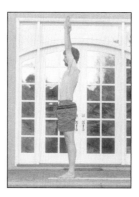

8b. Sun Salutations
pages 167–173

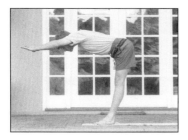

8c. Sun Salutations
pages 167–173

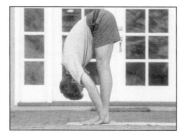

8d. Sun Salutations
pages 167–173

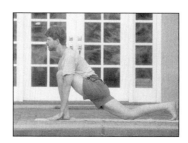

8e. Sun Salutations
pages 167–173

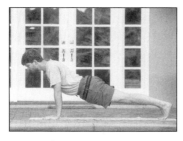

8f. Sun Salutations
pages 167–173

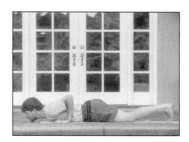

8g. Sun Salutations
pages 167–173

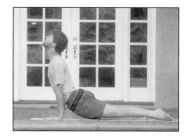

8h. Sun Salutations
pages 167–173

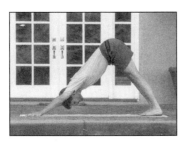

8i. Sun Salutations
pages 167–173

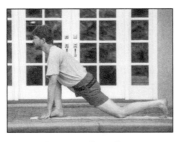

8j. Sun Salutations
pages 167–173

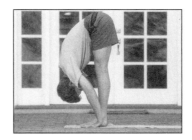

8k. Sun Salutations
pages 167–173

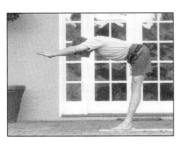

8l. Sun Salutations
pages 167–173

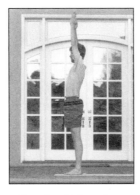

8m. Sun Salutations
pages 167–173

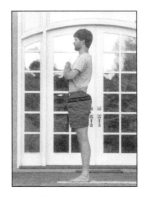

8n. Sun Salutations
pages 167–173

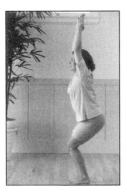

9. Zig Zag Pose
(Utkasana)
pages 75–76

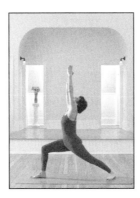

10. Warrior I
(Virabhadrasana I)
pages 140–141

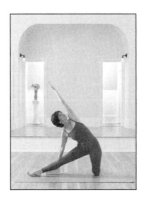

11. Gate Pose
(Parighasana)
pages 132–133

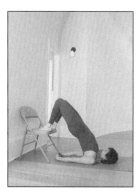

12. Bridge Pose
(Setu Bandha)
with chair
pages 84–86

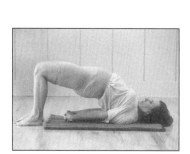

13. Bridge Pose
(Setu Bandha)
pages 84–86

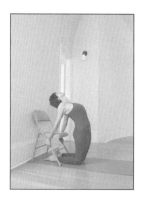

14. Camel Pose
with chair
(Ustrasana)
page 154

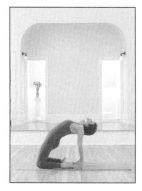

15. Camel Pose
(Ustrasana)
pages 124–125

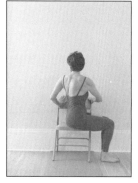

16. Chair Twist
(Chair Bharadvajasana)
page 155

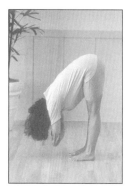

17. Standing
Forward Bend
(Uttanasana)
pages 81–82

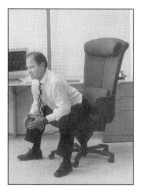

18a. Back and
Shoulder Release
pages 32–33

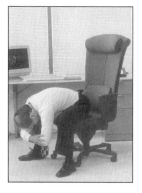

18b. Back and
Shoulder Release
pages 32–33

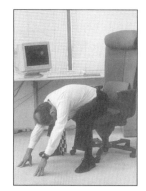

18c. Back and
Shoulder Release
pages 32–33

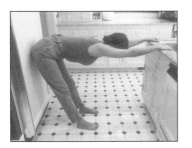 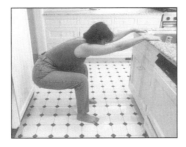 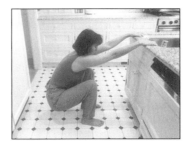

19a. Three-Part Pull
pages 202–204

19b. Three-Part Pull
pages 202–204

19c. Three-Part Pull
pages 202–204

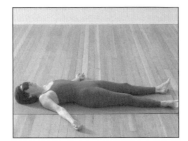

20. Relaxation
(Savasana)
pages 157–158

Friday
Forward Bends

Focus: These poses focus on the opportunity to surrender on all physical, mental and emotional levels. As we release into these forward bends, they teach us to move from the gross to the subtle, and from the active to the more peaceful and reflective state of mind.

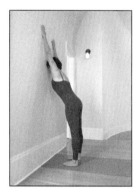

1. Wall Stretch
page 41

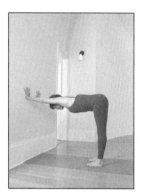

2. Right-Angled Wall Stretch
(Ardha Uttanasana)
pages 108–109

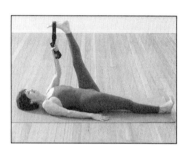

3a. Hamstring Stretch
(Supta Padangusthasana)
pages 126–128

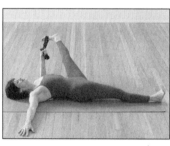

3b. Hamstring Stretch
(Supta Padangusthasana)
pages 126–128

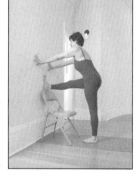

4a. Standing Hamstring Stretch & Inner Thigh Stretch
(Utthita Hasta Padangusthasana I & II)
pages 114–115

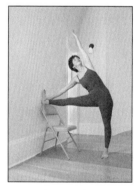

4b. Standing Hamstring Stretch & Inner Thigh Stretch
(Utthita Hasta Padangusthasana I & II)
pages 148–149

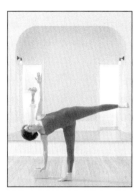

5. Half Moon Pose
(Ardha Chandrasana)
pages 134–137

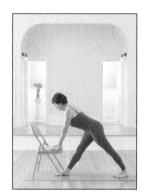

**6. One-legged
Hamstring Stretch
with chair**
(Parsvottanasana)
pages 141–143

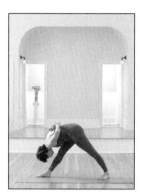

**7. One-Legged
Hamstring Stretch**
(Parsvottanasana)
pages 142–144

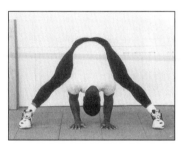

8. Wide-Angled Standing Pose
(Prasarita Padottanasana)
pages 115–117

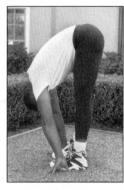

**9. Standing Forward
Bend**
(Uttanasana)
pages 117–118

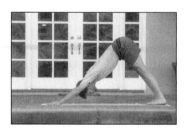

10. Downward Facing Dog
(Adho Mukha Svanasana)
pages 161–163

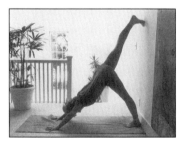

**11. Downward Facing Dog
with One Leg Up**
(Adho Mukha Svanasana)
pages 194–195

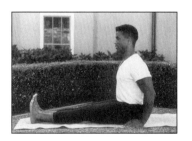

12. Staff Pose
(Dandasana)
pages 118–119

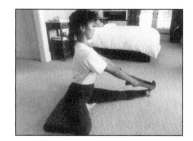

13. Head to Knee Pose
(Janusirsasana)
pages 183–185

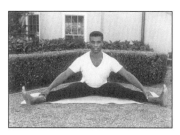

14. Wide-Angled Sitting Pose
(Upavistha Konasana)
pages 118–119

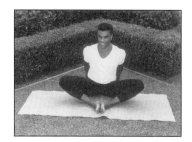

15. Bound Angle Pose
(Baddha Konasana)
pages 120–121

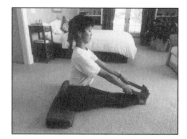

16. Full Forward Bend
(Paschimottanasana)
pages 185–186

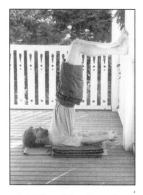

17. Shoulder Stand at Wall
(Salamba Sarvangasana)
pages 174–175

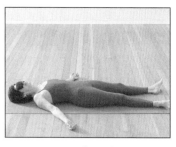

18. Relaxation
(Savasana)
pages 157–158

Saturday
Twists and Abdominals

Focus: These poses focus on the therapeutic application of twists and abdominal strengthening. The muscles and organs are squeezed, then released, to allow blood and nutrients to soak and spread into these areas, thereby bringing energy and vitality to the entire body.

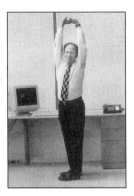

1. Gentle Twist
pages 25–26

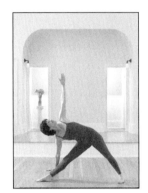

2. Chair Twist
(Chair Bharadvajasana)
page 155

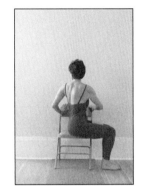

3. Triangle Pose
(Utthita Trikonasana)
pages 76–77

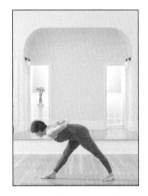

**4a. One-Legged
Hamstring Stretch**
(Parsvottanasana)
pages 142–144

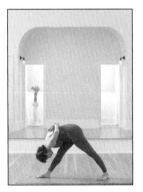

**4b. One-Legged
Hamstring Stretch**
(Parsvottanasana)
pages 142–144

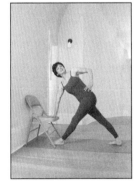

5. Revolved Triangle
*(Parivritta
Trikonasana)*
pages 144–146

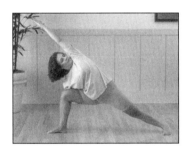

6. Right-Angled Side Stretch
(Utthita Parsvakonasana)
pages 79–81

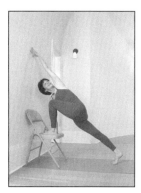

7. Revolved Right-Angled Side Stretch
(Parivritta Parsvakonasana)
pages 146–148

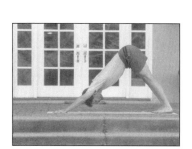

8. Downward Facing Dog
(Adho Mukha Svanasana)
pages 161–163

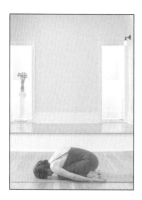

9. Child's Pose
pages 53 and 125

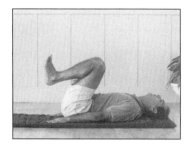

10a. Knee to Chest Abdominal
pages 96–98

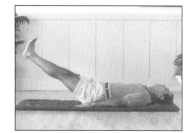

10b. Knee to Chest Abdominal
pages 96–98

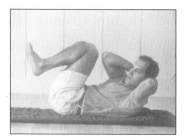

11. Abdominal Cross Overs
pages 98–100

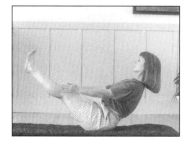

12. Complete Boat Pose
(Paripurna Navasana)
pages 101–102

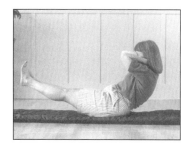

13. Half Boat Pose
(Ardha Navasana)
pages 102–103

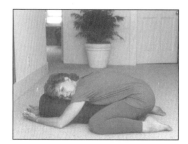

14. Child's Pose on a Bolster
pages 196–197

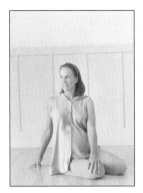

15. Sitting Twist
(Bharadvajasana)
page 191

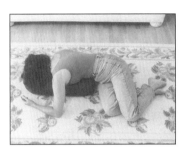

16. Twist facing Bolster
(Supta Bharadvajasana)
pages 213–214

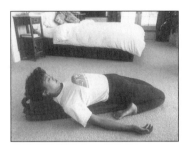

17. Reclined Hero
(Supta Virasana)
pages 181-183

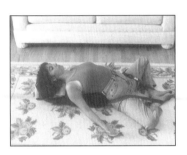

**18. Reclined Bound
Angle Pose**
(Supta Baddha Konasana)
pages 210–211

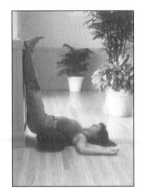

**19. Lazy Shoulder
Stand**
(Viparita Karani)
pages 212–213

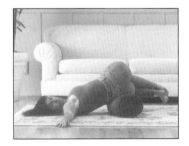

20. Twist on Bolster
(Jatara Parivartanasana)
pages 207–208

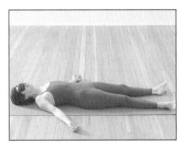

21. Relaxation
(Savasana)
pages 157–158

A Balanced Class

Focus: These poses focus on a well-rounded practice to create balance in one's life as well as on the mat. This practice helps you find flexibility with strength, a feeling of being energized yet calm, and gaining a state of stability with ease.

A favorite quote by Guru Maya is: "Remain in the state of tranquility and resist the temptation to struggle." May these poses help you with gaining that balance.

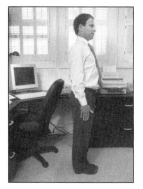
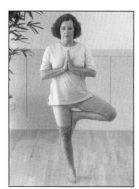
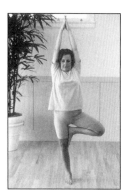
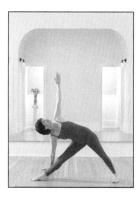

1. Palm Tree Pose
(Tadasana)
pages 18–19

2a. Tree Pose
(Vrksasana)
pages 74–75

2b. Tree Pose
(Vrksasana)
pages 74–75

3. Triange Pose
(Trikonasana)
pages 76–77

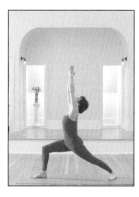
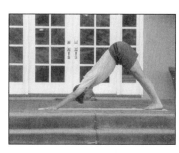
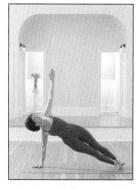

4. Warrior I
(Virabhadrasana I)
pages 140–141

5. Downward Facing Dog
(Adho Mukha Svanasana)
pages 161–163

6. Arm Balance and Back Strengthener
(Vasisthasana)
pages 151–153

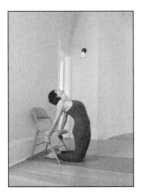

**7. Camel Pose
with chair**
(Ustrasana)
page 154

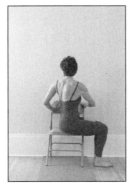

8. Chair Twist
*(Chair
Bharadvajasana)*
page 155

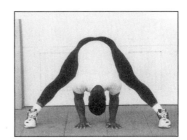

9. Wide-Angled Standing Pose
(Prasarita Padottanasana)
pages 115–117

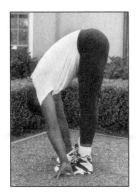

**10. Standing Forward
Bend**
(Uttanasana)
pages 117–118

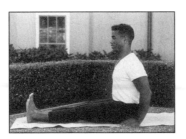

11. Staff Pose
(Dandasana)
pages 118–119

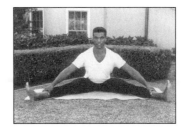

12. Wide-Angled Sitting Pose
(Upavista Konasana)
pages 118–119

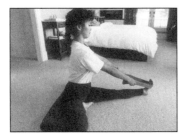

13. Head to Knee Pose
(Janusirsasana)
pages 183–185

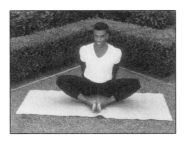

14. Bound Angle Pose
(Baddha Konasana)
pages 120–121

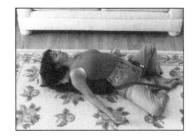

15. Reclined Bound Angle Pose
(Supta Baddha Konasana)
pages 210–211

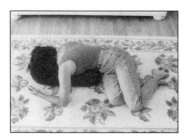

16. Twist facing Bolster
(Supta Bharadvajasana)
pages 213–214

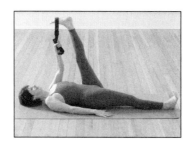

17a. Hamstring Stretch
(Supta Padangusthasana)
pages 126–128

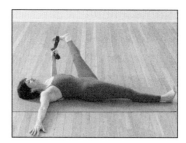

17b. Hamstring Stretch
(Supta Padangusthasana)
pages 126–128

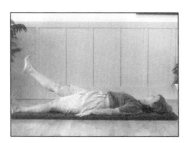

18. Leg Lifts
(Urdhva Prasarita Padasana)
pages 94–96

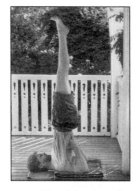

19. Shoulder Stand
*(Salamba
Sarvangasana)*
pages 174–177

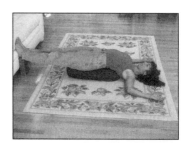

**20. Bridge on Bolster
Supported**
(Setu Bandha Sarvangasana)
pages 209–210

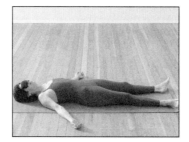

21. Relaxation
(Savasana)
pages 157–158

a f t e r w o r d

_____

If you are reading this book, we will assume that you want to enjoy life to the maximum. Now you have the tools to help yourself . . .

- Reduce stress
- Improve your health and well-being
- Increase your mental clarity
- Live life with more vitality

We have told you that yoga stretching will give you more energy and make you feel more alive. Elise is living proof. She has made yoga her life. What we have waited to tell you is why. Here is Elise's personal story:

"When I was fifteen, I was diagnosed by my physician with a severe scoliosis curve. The pain was debilitating. It was difficult for me to sit without having shooting pains up my back. Bracing and surgery were recommended. For a second opinion, I consulted an orthopedic surgeon. Since I was at the end of my adolescent growth, he suggested that I first try a regimen of exercise including swimming and yoga. So I took his advice and started swimming and began a life-long practice of yoga.

"I have practiced yoga almost every day. Not only has yoga changed my physical appearance, but practicing it has reduced my spinal curvature. This has required dedication and perseverance, but I am now essentially pain free and can lead a completely normal life.

"You do not have to have a life-threatening disease to get benefits from yoga stretching. We hope you have tried at least a few stretches and encourage you to put stretching into your life every day. Use the stretches that apply to your normal routine, and when your routine changes, find new stretches to match your new activities or new condition.

"We hope you will continue exploring a variety of the stretches we have offered you. And when you become familiar with a selection of them, you can create your own, individualized program."

Here are some final words of encouragement:

- Always begin with breath awareness

- Regular practice is important

- Don't set yourself up for failure and commit to do yoga for an unrealistic amount of time—commit to an amount of time that you feel you truly will do; you can always do more out of desire rather than commitment; better to start with a ten-minute practice and build up to twenty minutes rather than high expectations of an hour and then fail

- Set aside a regular time to practice; make an appointment with yourself and put that time you are going to do yoga in your appointment book; it is best if it is the same time each day so it becomes routine—mornings and evenings are best

- Start with your favorite poses and ones you are most familiar with, then you can move on to the ones you need

- To avoid injury, do not force the body beyond its capacity; play the edge, feeling the sensation, but not going beyond where the entire body tightens and you feel pain

- Routines are good but remember to listen to your body and do what feels appropriate for that day—know when to push and when to lighten up; learn to distinguish between excuses and real signals; it's easier said than done, but the more you practice, the easier it will become to distinguish between those two

- Be patient; remember, it took all those years to develop tension, so give a little time to letting that tension go

- Use yoga as a tool to improve your life, not to make you perfect

Life will always present us with challenges, whether it is a tight hamstring, or a tight timetable, or a tight situation. Let *Yoga* give you the strength and flexibility to handle the given moment, *anytime, anywhere*!

suggested resources

Yoga Connections

Yoga with Elise Miller

Go to Elise's websites for more information about her: http://www.ebmyoga.com and www.yogaforscoliosis.com

Magazines

Yoga Journal: 1-800-436-9642,
http://www.yogajournal.com

Yoga International: 1-800-253-6243,
http://www.yimag.com

Where to Find a Yoga Teacher Online:

http://www.iynaus.org
http://www/yogaalliance.com
http://www.yogajournal.com
http://www.yogateachersassoc.org

Equipment

Gaiam
http://www.gaiam.com

Tools for Yoga
http://www.toolsforyoga.net

Yoga Props
http://www.yogaprops.net

Hugger Mugger Yoga Products
http://www.huggermugger.com

Bheka Yoga Supplies
http://www.bheka.com

Yoga Mats
http://www.yogamats.com

bibliography

Iyengar, B. K. S. *Light On Pranayama*. New York, NY: Crossroad, 1981.

———. *Light On Yoga*. New York, NY: Schocken Books, 1966.

———. *Yoga: The Path to Holistic Health*. London: Dorling Kindersley, 2001.

Iyengar, Geeta S. *Yoga, A Gem for Women*. Palo Alto, CA: Timeless Books, 1990.

Silva, Mira & Shyam Mehta. *Yoga, The Iyengar Way*. New York, NY: Alfred Knopf, 1990.

index

---

contact

If you wish to contact the authors or would like more information about this book, please write to the authors in care of Llewellyn Worldwide and we will forward your request. The authors and publisher appreciate hearing from you and learning of your enjoyment of this book and how it has helped you. Llewellyn Worldwide cannot guarantee that every letter written to the authors can be answered, but all will be forwarded. Please write to:

Elise Browning Miller and Carol Blackman
℅ Llewellyn Worldwide
P.O. Box 64383, Dept. 0-7387-0635-3
St. Paul, MN 55164-0383, U.S.A.

Please enclose a self-addressed, stamped envelope for reply,
or $1.00 to cover costs.
If outside U.S.A., enclose international postal reply coupon.

Free Magazine

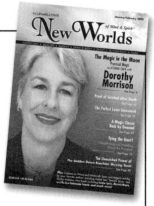

Read unique articles by Llewellyn authors, recommendations by experts, and information on new releases. To receive a **free** copy of Llewellyn's consumer magazine, *New Worlds of Mind & Spirit,* simply call 1-877-NEW-WRLD or visit our website at www.llewellyn.com and click on *New Worlds.*

☾ LLEWELLYN ORDERING INFORMATION

 Order Online:
Visit our website at www.llewellyn.com, select your books, and order them on our secure server.

 Order by Phone:
- Call toll-free within the U.S. at 1-877-NEW-WRLD (1-877-639-9753).
  Call toll-free within Canada at 1-866-NEW-WRLD (1-866-639-9753)
- We accept VISA, MasterCard, and American Express

 Order by Mail:
Send the full price of your order (MN residents add 7% sales tax) in U.S. funds, plus postage & handling to:

**Llewellyn Worldwide
P.O. Box 64383, Dept. 0-7387-0635-3
St. Paul, MN 55164-0383, U.S.A.**

Postage & Handling:

Standard (U.S., Mexico, & Canada). If your order is:
$49.99 and under, add $3.00
$50.00 and over, FREE STANDARD SHIPPING

AK, HI, PR: $15.00 for one book plus $1.00 for each additional book.

International Orders (airmail only):
$16.00 for one book plus $3.00 for each additional book

Orders are processed within 2 business days. Please allow for normal shipping time. Postage and handling rates subject to change.

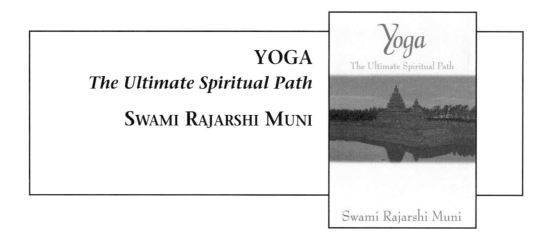

YOGA
The Ultimate Spiritual Path
SWAMI RAJARSHI MUNI

Yoga: The Ultimate Spiritual Path is a groundbreaking work for serious seekers and scholars about spontaneous yoga—the yoga of liberation. Instead of discussing the physical exercises or meditations usually understood to be yoga in the West, this book focuses on a proven process by which you can achieve liberation from the limitations of time and space, unlimited divine powers, and an immortal, physically perfect, divine body that is retained forever.

The sages who composed the ancient Indian scriptures achieved such a state—as have people of all religious traditions. How? Through the process of surrendering the body and mind to the spontaneous workings of the awakened life force: prana. Once prana is awakened, it works in its own amazing way to purify your physical and nonphysical body. Over time, all the bondage of karma is released, and you become fully liberated.

1-56718-441-3
224 pp., 7 ½ x 9 ⅛, illus.   **$14.95**

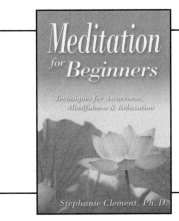

Meditation for Beginners
Techniques for Awareness, Mindfulness & Relaxation

STEPHANIE CLEMENT, PH.D.

Award Winner!

Break the barrier between your conscious and unconscious minds.

Perhaps the greatest boundary we set for ourselves is the one between the conscious and less conscious parts of our own minds. We all need a way to gain deeper understanding of what goes on inside our minds when we are awake, asleep, or just not paying attention. Meditation is one way to pay attention long enough to find out.

Meditation for Beginners explores many different ways to meditate—including kundalini yoga, walking meditation, dream meditation, tarot meditations, and healing meditation—and offers a step-by-step approach to meditation, with exercises that introduce you to the rich possibilities of this age-old spiritual practice. Improve concentration, relax your body quickly and easily, work with your natural healing ability, and enhance performance in sports and other activities. Just a few minutes each day is all that's needed.

0-7387-0203-X
264 pp., 5 ³/₁₆ x 8, illus. $12.95

To order, call 1-877-NEW-WRLD
Prices subject to change without notice